HERBAL ANTIVIRALS

This book is an essential guide to herbal Remedies for a beginner. Replace traditional medicine with self Herbalism.
Catherine White

Contents

CHAPTER1: MEDICAL HERBALISM, AN ART OF PRACTICE

Herbalism is an ancient mode of treatment, which was probably the first type of treatment used against ailments and illnesses related to a human being. The human body is unique, and you can say a masterpiece of God. It comprises hundreds of bones, muscles, and ligaments which support the interior of the body and form an exoskeleton. It also contains many organs that are devoted to performing a number of actions to regulate the normal homeostasis of the human body. Homeostasis is the balance of the human body, which is essential for its proper working. Without a proper homeostatic balance, our body is unable to perform any necessary actions that are essential for life. In the human body, there are many organs and organ systems; however, some of these organs are essential for the health of human life, which is called vital organs. Heart, lungs, kidneys, liver, and brain are some vital organs. Anything which can disturb the homeostasis between these organs can lead to major catastrophes, which can include the death of the human body.

It is essential to know the basic functions of the human body so that specific drugs or treatments can be proposed to treat the illnesses related to the human body. Without Herbal antivirals relevant knowledge, no treatment can benefit a human organ system, and it may cause many unwanted side effects. It is highly necessary to say that working with the human body is a complete art. Our bodies are made in an artistic fashion. Every system and subsystem of the human body is interconnected, and anything which can benefit or deteriorate a body's homeostasis can be detrimental. Infections such as viral, bacterial, or fungal can cause many disturbances in the average homeostatic balance of the body, so damaging effects of these infections are much fold. Many treatment strategies, such as herbal, allopathic, homeopathic, and others, are used to treat these infections. Every school of thought has its own philosophy behind treating human illness, and specific principles are followed in every unique category.

It is essential to discuss the herbalist school of thought in detail. Herbalism is by far the most historical type of medical treatment strategy implemented by nearly every era of the human race and in every country of the world. Herbalism is the use of herbs for therapeutic purposes and poses a deep relationship between man and plant. It is widely practiced by every human culture, race, or religion. Herbalism is the most natural type of medical treatment in which herbs are grown and used to reduce the risks associated with herbs. A wide variety of different methods are implicated in using herbs for therapeutic purposes. Tinctures, solutions, grains, oils, and many other forms of herbs are used as a medication to treat nearly every system of the human body.

A herbalist is a person who grows, prepares, and uses herbs to treat the illnesses related to the human mind, body, and spirit. Herbalism has its basis on holistic pharma in which physical, emotional, and spiritual aspects of the human body are treated instead of just treating the cause. It is very different than homeopathy, allopathy (modern medicine), and other types of medical schools in treating human illnesses.

The herbalism is actually the pythotherapy in medical terminology in which plants are used to the mind, body, and spirit of a human being. It is a branch of holistic medicine in which specific herbs are used to treat multiple illnesses and conditions. It is comprised of the principle and practice of art and medicine to create a system of treatment. Nearly any condition which can be treated by allopath, homeopathy or other medicine systems can also be treated by herbal medicine. The benefits hidden in plants can affect the human physiological responses, and thus, any disturbances in them can also be treated by using plants as a medicine. Holistic medicine is evolving these days, and its roots are getting stronger day by day. Nearly every country of the world is using a holistic approach to medicine in every medical field. This shift of paradigm is not new to humankind, and it has historical grounds as well.

WHO is the official body which is responsible for defining the standard definitions related to medical and health. The definition of WHO about health involves the spiritual and mental aspects along with the physical integration of a human being, and it forces the practitioner to treat the human as a whole. A system of self-healing strategy is also an equally important concept in pythotherapy and holistic medicine. Hippocratic Oath also guides the herbalist to use strategies to treat human-being as a whole. A medical practitioner can be a Doctor or herbal medicine, osteopath, physician, or a qualified nurse who can use alternative therapies that are in the domain of holistic medicine and Herbal antivirals, a strong research background. It is of great importance to discuss the regulations and roles of medical herbalism practitioners who can use a holistic approach to treat patients. Nature greatly assists the philosophy and practice of a medical herbalism expert. The healing strategy used by a medical herbalist is called ecological healing because it uses plants and the ecological environment for healing of a condition.

The high strength of herbalism expert is the integration of traditional philosophies of healing with modern day scope of practice. Medical herbalism is very simple and highly complex at the same time. It is merely that a patient can get the maximum benefit of a weed by just growing it in his/her backyard and chewing it or drinking the dissolved solution. The complexities lie in the fundamental biochemical and pharmacological aspects of a herb using as a treatment of choice. The self-healing strategy used by a medical herbalist is to introduce a patient about a specific herb and providing him knowledge of proper uses and benefits of that specific herb. He/she makes the patient eligible to grow his/her own weed or herb and thus, provides a higher degree of autonomy to the patient. From a seed to a complete plant, a patient seeks close attachment with the growth of that plant, and thus, the benefits on the mind, body, and spirit of a patient introduced by the plant are many folds. In medical herbalism practice, a properly educated patient works in close coordination with a plant that not only cures his/her physical illnesses but also helps in experience a whole new life, from a seed to a full-grown plant.

A plant is a living entity that breaths, exchanges gases, grows while consuming the nutrition, and dies when depletion of nutrients occurs. Life and death are very similar as experienced by the human. So, this experience is highly crucial for a herbalist to know the basic principles of personal healing. An educated patient who experiences this phenomenon by himself can understand the art of living in a broader vision, and a much deeper attachment with the plant can also be obtained. This fantastic interaction affects the physiological responses occurring in mind, body, and spirit of humans, and thus, complete health in the context of physical, emotional, and spiritual wellbeing can be achieved by a herbalist easier than other non-natural medical philosophies. A person should know what is happing behind a specific healing process so that the complexities of human nature can be well understood and fewer chances of getting side effects. As a herbalism expert, it is essential to know the basic properties of a herb/plant. It is highly essential to know the biological and spiritual aspects of a human body so that the maximum impacts of herbs can be obtained by using specific plants and herbs.

Another important aspect of herbalism practice is to use the plant as a source of deep emotional attachment so that it can be grown in full capacities with compassion and care. A herbalist should know how to grow a specific herb/plant in multiple environments and soil conditions, which can be ideal for the maximum growth of a plant. This book will cover all these necessary steps of herbalism philosophy in the easiest possible ways so that new readers and fresh herbalism students can find the fundamental essence of herbalism.

Art of practice:

In herbalism school of thought, the underlying philosophy behind a treatment methodology is to follow a holism technique. A person should be treated as a whole rather than treating his/her symptoms. In holism philosophy, mind, body, and spirit are treated in close connection so that a complete form of health and wellness is achieved. A herbalist prepares land for the sowing of seeds of specific herbs, Provides water and takes care of that seed, observes the growth of a plant in close coordination, and provides a suitable environment for its maturity. All these steps are essential in making a connection between herbalists and his/her herbs. A herbalist is a doctor who treats a human being for his/her illnesses. The method used by a herbalist to treat illnesses is by using the medicinal benefits of herbs. So he/she acts as a vital bridge between the patient and herbs. So, the responsibility of a herbalist is two folds as compared to those doctors who treat a person by artificial use of medicine. A herbalist has to take care of humans and also herbs because both are living beings. Moreover, he/she has to take care of those birds, flies, and insects to which his herbal garden acts as a habitat. So it is easier to achieve kindness, care, and compassion for a herbalist for every living being he/she is in coordination with, and it will help him to achieve a heart of a humanist.

Herbalism is based on science, and scientific principles are mostly followed in herbalism practice to ensure high-quality, evidence-based practice. Scientific literature is enough to support the use of herbalism in treating human illnesses, but unfortunately, enough work is not done yet to prove it as a treatment of choice as compared to modern herbal medicine. It is a sole responsibility for every herbalist to publish scientific papers of his/her work to validate the effectiveness of herbalism. However, the WHO considers the independent practice of herbalists. WHO is the official body which is responsible for defining the standard definitions related to medical and health. The definition of WHO about health involves the spiritual and mental aspects along with the physical integration of a human being, and it forces the practitioner to treat the human as a whole. Due to this scientific and evidence-based practice, a herbalist essentially has the mind of a scientist.

The herbalist is a bridge between his plants and a human being to whom he provides medicinal benefits. He uses his hands to sow a seed in prepared land. His hands water the seed and take care of a newly growing plant. By using his hands, a herbalist handpicks the essential herbs, and after quality testing, herbal medicine is prepared in its most effective form to treat human illnesses. So, in this regard, we can say that it is pure art to treat in the context of herbalism philosophy. From growing plants to making a diagnosis and providing essential medicines to a specific human pathology, every step involves an artistic approach. So, it is essential to say that a herbalist also has the hands of artists. These characteristics make a herbalist eligible to treat human illnesses in the best possible ways.

To conclude the art of practice in the domain of herbalism, it is essential to say that a herbalist is a person who has the brain of a scientist, heart of a humanist, and mind of an artist. In short, a herbalist is a complete package, and to master this art of practice; it takes years of experience in the field of kindness, compassion, and science. A high-quality herbalist must possess a broad spectrum of knowledge in the field of botany and zoology, specifically human medicine.

CHAPTER2: HISTORY OF MEDICAL HERBALISM IN FIGHTING INFECTIONS

In today's tale, herbal medicine against infections is one of the most popular natural products being used by every age group, and social as well as print media is widely advertising its benefits. Still, this era is not the origin of apple herbs. National apple museum has conducted a critical historical survey about the background and advancements in herbal medicine against infection history. The first evidence of apple trees was found in Egyptian culture, and they were cultivated at the bank of Neil River. The literature is not complete to build a consensus that herbs were used in Egyptian civilization, but it is clear that they were very fond of beer even they were the first one who introduced it. So, it can be possible that they did enjoy the taste of herbal medicine against infections. However, history shows that once the drink was introduced, it spread at a swift pace over different zones of the globe, much like we are observing it today. In 55 B.C. after the arrival of Roman in British waters, they found locals enjoying a traditional herbs-like drink, which appealed to them too, and soon, it was being considered as one of their favorite beverages. So, this beverage, with small changes in the recipe, was introduced in the Roman Empire and then to Europe. It was the most popular drink of Germanic heritage, and they added it to the Normans. When Normans defeated the British Empire in the 9th century, they brought the word "herbs" into the English dictionary.

After Europe and the Mediterranean region, this herbal medicine against infections found its way to the earliest colonies. It was tough for European colonies to cultivate barley and grains for the production of beer, so they considered the herbs as the best alternative because apple trees were easy to grow on British lands. That was the course of discovery of herbal medicine against infections by the very dear America of Columbus. They enjoyed the drink, and it was boozy at the time and very different than the brown and sweet drink available. Herbal medicine against infections was used as a shield to save them during the chilling winter season. A legendry apple farmer, Johnny Appleseed, introduced a less alcoholic version, which was safer to use by the children.

There was a lag period in the American history of herbal medicine against infections when the Europeans and Germans settled in the Midwest and found it friendly to produce beer from barley and grains, so the use of herbal medicine against infections declined. Even, there was a prohibition period in American history when all the American herbalists were forcedly stopped from producing herbs, and this prohibition lasted for decades. The good thing is good, and herbs began to merge again, and it was the most popular energy booster during the winters.

The first written document about herbal medicine in Chinese is almost 5000 years old. Traditional Chinese medicine is unique in the use of terminologies like ying-yang and ashi points. Traditional Chinese ideology about medicine also used herbs as a fundamental source of healing, and this philosophy considers human as an evolving and dynamic nature which can self-heal if provided with the right environment. According to this theory, a dynamic balance between matter and energy is crucial to seek the complete form of health and wellbeing. The use of the healing capacities of nature to cure illnesses and self-healing is an essential term in traditional Chinese medicine. The term is also used by herbalism and other natural schools of medical treatment. Meridians were the terms used along with ashi points in Chinese medicine according to which energy can be trapped in these points (ashi points), and constant flow of meridians (energy) is essential for the complete health of a human being. Along with acupuncture and cupping therapy, herbal use of medicine was the most critical aspect of Chinese medicine. A large variety of herbs were utilized by ancient Chinese doctors to cure the imbalances between matter and energy, which were thought of as an essential basis of illnesses in human bodies. Western modern medicine is entirely different from the ancient Chinese system of medicine because in the western system, the only focus of interest is the matter, and energies are heavily neglected in modern western medicine because it can't be seen or calculated.

The oldest documents are available on herbal medicine Herbal antivirals origin in India in which ayurvedic medicine was used as a base of the health system. This system is solely comprised of using herbs as a base of the health and integrity of the human body. Pandits and Swamis of Indian culture were thought to be the medical practitioners as well as the religious bodies who could cure the human illnesses of physical, emotional, or spiritual nature. Herbs were always an essential component of traditional Indian medicine. These herbs were used in multiple forms to cure a variety of diseases. Some herbs were also used for magic and spiritual purposes. Indian traditional medical system is not entirely dead and is being practiced in India, as well as it is widely known to other countries during modern times too. The lively nature of this system which makes it fit even after thousands of year is because the natural sources of treatment which can never die till the Day of Judgment.

The culture at the bank of Neil is nearly 8000 years old. Along with the spectacular pyramids of Egypt, this culture also had amazing medical backgrounds. Herbs were considered as the most important remedies to cure human illness as well as in magic. The pharaoh of Egypt used special herbs to enhance their sexual and physical powers, as well as magic, had a strong base in Egyptian culture. Herbs had a crucial part in religious ceremonies and cultural events. The proofs of herbs used in medicine, as well as other aspects, can be seen through the walls of the great pyramids.

Islam is one of the most followed religions in the world, and its history is nearly 1400 years old. In the Islamic system of medicine, the word Tibb was used, and Tabib was the doctor who was eligible to practice medicine. Avicenna is known as the father of biology, who was a Muslim scientist of the same era. There are thousands of books and proofs in Islamic literature that show that the traditional Islamic system of medicine was based on herbal medicine. Herbs were used in calculated doses to treated illnesses related to human bodies. Some herbs were used for aromatherapy and perfumes as Arabic culture is rich in the use of aroma called It, which is based on herbs.

Herbal antivirals; a debate on current pandemic:

Herbal antivirals belong to a particular class of herbal medicine, which involves the use of herbal medicine against viruses. Medical science is continuously evolving and considering the newest and more effective treatments for common illnesses and even for more deadly and severe infections, which are causing massive loss to human-being all over the globe. The source of transmission and mode of spread of viruses and bacteria, which cause some deadly infections, is through the air, through the animal source, from one infected person to another healthy individual either by touching or through droplets. Some of these airborne infections are simple, yet others are highly complicated. The cause of the transmission of these diseases can be preventable. However, some infections don't occur. These infections don't have a good prognosis and poor treatment options. The only source to fight with these deadly infections is to prevent them by utilizing robust preventive measures and safety precautions. The only source to avoid getting this infection is to you all the preventive measures because; prevention is more helpful in saving lives from this disease. These airborne infections are highly transmissible and thus can affect a vast population within minimum time, and even some of these infections can lead to global pandemics. No industry is spared from getting affected very severely from this disease, and even the healthcare supplies of regular use Herbal antivirals suffered a lot. The most crucial line of prevention against the crown-type virus is alcohol-based hand sanitizer and herbal antivirals. Unfortunately, the proper preventive tools and measures require worldwide production and consumption, which means if more human population affects by these airborne viruses, it may cause lockdowns and shut down production companies, which can lead to catastrophic effects. These severe emergencies caused by airborne infections can lead to disturbed financial map all over the world, which affects the supply of preventive item supplies in the world mainly, in countries which are down the poverty line. So, in time of extreme medical emergency and a severe shortage of healthcare supplies, any tips or tricks which can be utilized to produce these essential preventive tools at home should be utilized. This book will discuss the easiest ways to prepare different types of herbal antivirals at home to prevent the PANDEMICS infection during the frightening period of lockdown and isolation in which these crucial medical supplies are not available in the needed quantity. The most common and historical pandemics in which Herbal antivirals infected the entire world in the past decades are cholera, tuberculosis, influenza virus, and many others. The underlying mechanism of the spread of these infections is the transfer through air and water droplets, which are present in the air. This is the reason that these infections are called airborne type. Some of these airborne infections affect nearly 2 million people every day around the globe. So, constant preventions of these viruses and bacteria should be utilized to avoid catastrophic results. High-quality homemade face mask with or without pocket is the best available preventive tool for these airborne infections

Chosen benefits of herbal antivirals during pandemics:

During pandemics, when every country suffers lockdowns and quarantine issues, many crucial health supplies become extinct from the market. This leads to a global human crisis in that scenario. Homemade herbal antivirals play a very crucial role in maintaining the crucial health supply against these bacteria and viruses. Herbal medicines made from amla, neem, and many other natural sources are highly beneficial in the fight against deadly microorganisms. Regular and proper use of these homemade herbal antivirals is highly essential to protect against these infections, which can cause catastrophic effects.

CHAPTER3: HERBAL ANTIVIRALS VS MODERN MEDICINE

Herbal medicine is used to treat nearly all types of infections and diseases. It is one of the oldest forms of treatment strategy used for treating human illnesses. It is essential to know that in nearly every civilization, herbal medicine used as a treatment of choice for common and uncommon diseases to human beings. Some civilizations also used herbal medicine as a source of green magic. Some black magic also involved the use of herbs. In today's tale, herbal medicine is one of the most popular natural products being used by every age group, and social as well as print media is widely advertising its benefits. Still, this era is not the origin of herbs. National apple museum has conducted a critical historical survey about the background and advancements in herbal medicine history. The first evidence of apple trees was found in Egyptian culture, and they were cultivated at the bank of Neil River. The literature is not complete to build a consensus that herbs were used in Egyptian civilization, but it is clear that they were very fond of beer even they were the first one who introduced it. So, it can be possible that they did enjoy the taste of herbal medicine. However, history shows that once the drink was introduced, it spread at a swift pace over different zones of the globe, much like we are observing it today. In 55 B.C. after the arrival of Roman in British waters, they found locals enjoying a traditional cider-like drink, which appealed to them too, and soon, it was being considered as one of their favorite beverages. So, this beverage, with small changes in the recipe, was introduced in the Roman Empire and then to Europe. It was the most popular drink of Germanic heritage, and they added it to the Normans. When Normans defeated the British Empire in the 9th century, they brought the word "cider" into the English dictionary.

After Europe and the Mediterranean region, this herbal medicine found its way to the earliest colonies. It was tough for European colonies to cultivate barley and grains for the production of beer, so they considered the cider as the best alternative because apple trees were easy to grow on British lands. That was the course of discovery of herbal medicine by the very dear America of Columbus. They enjoyed the drink, and it was boozy at the time and very different than the brown and sweet drink available. Herbal medicine was used as a shield to save them during the chilling winter season. A legendry apple farmer, Johnny Appleseed, introduced a less alcoholic version, which was safer to use by the children.

There was a lag period in the American history of herbal medicine when the Europeans and Germans settled in the Midwest and found it friendly to produce beer from barley and grains, so the use of herbal medicine declined. Even, there was a prohibition period in American history when all the American cideries were forcedly stopped from producing cider, and this prohibition lasted for decades. The good thing is good, and cider began to merge again, and it was the most popular energy booster during the winters.

The history of modern medicine is also very unique. It gained popularity in the last decades of the 20th century. However, much work is done during the 21st century to build a consensus that modern medicine is by the most effective type of treatment used for human illnesses. The reason for this development is the use of medical research. Much work is done by the practitioners of modern medicine in the field of medical research, which is highly lagging among herbal medicine. There are a lot of controversies among the use of modern medicine to downfall another school of thought. However, it is not a place to discuss this point here. The most significant difference between modern and herbal medicine is the use of nature. Modern medicine uses synthetic, artificial, and laboratory-made salts to get the work done in preparation for common salts for medicine. However, medical herbalism is an old school using a hundred percent of nature in the preparation of herbal medicine.

In the next subheadings, some essential components of herbal medicine are discussed in detail.

Analyzing techniques for herbal medicine:

Herbs are used by herbalists to cure human illnesses in multiple forms and remedies. The quality control of herbs, as well as the underlying processes imposed by these herbs to cure the diseases, is highly essential to understand to avoid risks and dangers related to toxicity and overdose. Many other factors are also used to assess the quality of a herb.

Organoleptic analysis:

The use of human organs or, more specifically, the human senses to assess something is called the organoleptic analysis. Human being has five senses, i.e., smell, sight, taste, touch, and hearing. The first four senses are crucial to assess the quality of a herb. It will give a rough idea about the freshness and odor of a herb. The quality of the herb is organoleptic analysis is not sufficient until further analysis is carried out to confirm the safety issues related to herbs.

Microscopic analysis:

The use of a microscope becomes essential when the herb is assessed in its powdered form. Not every herb is fresh and safe for human use, and it can also contain some harmful pollens, fungi, algae, bacteria, and viruses. Microscopic analysis confirms the presence or absence of these microorganisms in powdered herbs.

Physical analysis:

Crude nature, melting point, shape, texture, color, and weight are some essential aspects of a herb that can be assessed by carrying out a physical analysis of herbs. It is essential because it gives a specific private label to a herb about its dosage and texture.

Chemical analysis:

Chemical analysis is essential to know about the chemistry of a herb. It is essential to carry out a chemical analysis because it will give essential ideas about the toxicity, dosage, or uses of a herb. Amino acid content, fats, carbohydrates, vitamins, minerals, alkaloids, acids, poisons, and many other critical chemical aspects of a herb can only be found by carrying out specific chemical analysis. It is by far the most important type of analysis related to quality control ad usage of a herb and can only be carried out by experts. Different types of chromatography (gas, liquid, weight) are used to know about the specific chemical nature of a herb. An herbalist must seek professional help to carry out these chemical analyses.

Biological analysis:

Another critical analysis that shows the specific biological characteristics of a herb as well as to assess the impacts of herbs on biological responses of the body. The biological analysis encompasses the specific measures to calculate the proper dosage of a herb. It can be a hit and trial method, and cadaver studies are carried out in which animals are used first to assess the specific impacts of a calculated dose of the herb in order to get the right idea about its impact on the human body. Another use of biological analysis is to measure the level of toxicity that can be occurred by overdosing the herb. It can also lead to catastrophic impacts when a dose is given above a standard dose. Toxicology is the study of toxicity related to any compound which is introduced in the human body. From a broader perspective, biological analysis is also used to check specific impacts of a herb on specific organ systems/systems in the human body so that a complete code can be formulated specifying the uses and dosage of a herb to benefit the human body.

Mode of actions and administration for herbal medicines:

Herbal medicine is made up of herbs, which contain medicinal benefits. The use of herbal medicine is very traditional; however, with the advancement of scientific methodologies and research, the use of herbal medicine is in context with a specific mode of actions within the human body. For example, if we want to treat infection within the lungs, applying for herbal medicine on the skin will be a bad idea. However, if we drink herbal drinks or consume drops of herbal tinctures, the medicine can directly be supplied into the lung fields where its medicinal impacts can provide amazing benefits against deadly viral and bacterial infections. So, it is highly essential to throw light on the specific mode of actions used in herbal medicine.

Herbal medicine used orally:

Tinctures, drops, teas, and decoction are used as oral routes for the administration of herbal drugs in the body. These forms of medicine are usually diluted in water or alcohol, and a fraction of herbal extract or pure herb is used to form oral formulations of herbal medicine. Tea is well known and probably the most consumed beverage in the world. The use of this herb for medicinal purposes is well known and has a strong research background. Black tea requires the essential and partial fermentation process of the tea leaves. However, green tea doesn't require these kinds of fermentation and can be produced through the process of steaming the leaves. This process reduces the oxidation capacities of enzymes present in tea leaves, and the preservation of polyphenol is achieved through this process. It is interesting to know that Polyphenols belong to a family of flavonoids which are present 30-40 percent of the total weight in dried green tea leaves. Camellia sinensis is a known name of dried and unfermented green tea leaves. It has a property to reduce bacterial and viral activities in the body. It is also essential in lowering down the increased concentration of lipids in the blood. The potency of green tea to lower down the blood cholesterol level is excellent, and thus it is a beverage of choice to reduce some extra pounds from the body. It is a potent anti-lipidemic agent. Its antioxidant benefits make it a perfect choice to detoxify the liver, kidneys, intestine, stomach, and skin. Its detoxifying and lipid-lowering benefits make it a perfect choice as a natural healer. The scientific base behind green tea is solid, and it is used in traditional as well as modern medicine as a natural source to treat many common illnesses of the human body. It is a super herb in holism, and the benefits of this herb are beyond the capacity of this essential book on holism.

Dosing of tea depends upon different factors and situations. When used in acute disorders and illnesses, the current complaint guides the dosage. Acute conditions may require multiple doses per day as compared to chronic doses, which require fewer doses for a prolonged time. Herbal medicine incorporates dosage according to the individual needs of a person rather than just treating symptoms with predetermined dosing strategies. It is not essential to stick with a specific pattern of dosing, and it can vary according to personal needs and interests, which is not practice when it comes to western allopathic medicine.

Teas are made from the specific plants of the tea family, and leaves of tea plants are mostly used in this process. However, other parts, such as flowers, can also be used. It can be made from dried or fresh parts of tea making plants, and the servings per day can vary from 2-6 doses depending upon personal needs and tolerance. Sampling mixing the leaves of tea plants in a hot water cup and mixing with honey can provide thousands of health benefits, or it can be made by proper boiling and adding milk, etc. which is called actual fermentation of tea such as black tea.

Tea can be made from handpicked leaves of tea plant grown in self botanic gardens, or it can be made from pre-designed herbal tea bags for convenience. When aromatic tea sources such as rosemary are used, its steam can also provide a face freshening treatment, which is a common practice in many western and Indian ayurvedic beauty treatments. Artificial or natural sweeteners such as honey can be used for adding more flavor to herbal teas. Stevia teas are naturally lovely in taste. Take a pinch of stevia tea, cool it in open-air then put it in a freezer bag. Then these bags can be put flat in freezers. When hit, a layer of frozen stevia tea can be break into ice chips, which can be used in other drinks to sweeten them as well as many benefits of stevia tea can be obtained through this process in regular drinks.

Decoctions are widely used sources of herbal medicine in herbalism. When roots or barks of plants contain medicinal benefits, it is hard to obtain extracts from these hard parts of plants, such as willow bark. Decoctions are great ways when the extraction of herbal medicine is required from these hard parts of plants. To obtain this, simmer the herb in hot water pan for at least twelve to thirty minutes on low flame. 1:32 ratio is essential to obtain decoctions from the herbs. A commonly used recipe involves 30 grams of herb and 1000ml of water.

Teas and decoctions are widely used as a herbal source of medicine preparation, and the reason behind using them on a wide-scale is easy to use properties. Just sipping through the cup is all it requires to administer the medicine inside the body. Even rinses and gargles can also be made from these two sources to relieve symptoms related to mouth and throat diseases. Popsicles can be made from a variety of sources, and it is an excellent source of reducing inflammation and pain related to the oral mucosa. Another benefit of popsicle is its incredible taste and ease of use. Ice cubes are a fantastic source of herbal delivery, and they are straightforward to administer. It can be made from teas and decoctions as well. Liquid herbal medicine can be frozen after boiling and rapid cooling, a process called thawing. It also contains pain-relieving benefits, which are very specific with cold therapy. If we add sticks inside ice cubes, they can easily be turned into homemade sweet popsicles. This form of administration is highly famous among children. The ice bags and trays should be labeled accordingly to avoid issues.

The basic model of action for using a herbal medicine orally is to provide an entry route of liquid medicine inside the body through the oral cavity. This is the most effective mode of administration in dental herbalism to treat illnesses related to gums, teeth, and oral mucosa. Teas and decoctions, when used, directly baths the structures inside the oral cavity, and absorptions of medicinal substances take place right in the oral mucosa. Sometimes, the oral route is also used to treat infections related to ear, nose, and throat because these structures Herbal antivirals same opening in the oral cavity and any disease present in one of these structures can pass through other structures as well. So, it is a highly important route for the administration of herbal medicine. The oral route is also used to treat the illnesses present in food pipes such as heartburns, digestive issues, and gastroesophageal reflux diseases. Illnesses present in the stomachs such as stomach ulcers and increased secretion of stomach acid are also controlled by taking herbal medicine orally. Illnesses present in the liver, pancreas, gallbladder, and intestines are also covered through the administration of herbal medicine in the body via the oral route. So it is the most crucial route to treat the organs related disorders as well as diseases in the oral mucosa.

Tinctures are drops of herbs in liquid form, which are combined in 80-95% of the alcohol base. The most crucial benefit of this type of administration is the very long preservation period of medicine achieved by adding alcohol into it. It is such a diluted form of medicine that hardly any side effect can occur. This is the sole reason that homeopaths used these types of tinctures from centuries to administer drugs in human bodies. The tincture can be prepared by mixing herb into wine, vodka, or rum. A more diluted media such as herbal medicine or glycerine can also be used to achieve these benefits. Alcohol-free media can also be used to make tinctures of very diluted quality for those who don't like alcohol to get ingested. Tinctures can be prepared in homes as well as they can also be available in markets. However, the best practice is to make it at home because it doesn't require any special treatment to prepare all these effective tinctures at home. Lany herbalists are famous for making their own tinctures. Raw alcohol is best to make tinctures rather than flavored vodka or rum so that the maximum benefits of herbs can be preserved. Flavoring is also rich in dirty surfers, which are not the right choice for medicinal purposes. Grain alcohol is the most popular type of alcohol used by herbalists to achieve the preparation of the highest quality tinctures. Vodka and grain are very different because they are made from very different sources. Twenty percent net alcohol should be used when the dried herb is made, and 40% of alcohol can be mixed with the fresh herb to ensure proper mixture and administration without side effects.

Willow bark is known to Herbal antivirals high tannin concentration, and thus adding a few amounts of glycerin can be a smart idea for extracting maximum concentration of herb. A tincture is nothing when inferior ingredients are used. Alcohol is just a base in it; however, the medicinal benefits of a tincture can only be achieved from using proper herbs only. A perfect ratio is 1:5, that is 1 part alcohol with five parts of herbs to ensure more concentration of herb in a tincture. This guide is a critical ad accepted in herbalist society all over the world. In the case of yarrow, we make an alcohol-based. Yarrow or other types of tannin-containing herbs can be mixed with glycerine and alcohol to extract the medicinal benefits from them properly. The next stage is to put the solution in a dark room while keeping the solution in a tight jar for more than three weeks. A proper shaking the jar every week can also promote proper extraction of the herbal medicinal benefits.

The use of tea and decoction, along with water, can also be applied while making an alcohol free tincture. The final step of tincturing is to stain the solution. The solution is called menstruum, which, while stained, is called a tincture. It is essential to label the jar with the proper name for identification purposes.

Herbal medicine used on the skin:

Herbal medicines are also applied as ointments and creams as well as in the form of wash clothes, poultices, and compresses. Washcloths are indeed a great source to get bathed on the bed. They can be used on a critically ill patient who cannot survive an active bath. In this comfortable way, medicine can easily be applied to the skin, and thus it can be transferred in a deeper area of the body through diffusion. Washcloths can be warm by using hot infusions of medicine when specific impacts of heating are needed, or they can be cold when benefits of cold are needed. It all depends upon personal choice as well as symptoms of illnesses. For acute injuries, for example, brushing and combat sports fights, cold washcloths with specific benefits of ice and anti-inflammatory medicine can be a smart choice to limit swelling and bruising as well as impeding bleeding from fresh wounds. Cold also has anesthetic properties, which make it a natural pain killer.

When used warm, washcloths can stimulate blood flow due to vasodilatory effects as well as a soothing response of the body can also be obtained.

Compresses are warm medicinal pastes which are formed from many potent herbs. It is a very traditional technique, which is also caller "Marham" in Arabic, and it is the most used technique in Indian ayurvedic as well. Warm herbs in the form of compresses can stay longer than washcloths on the skin and can be a great source of constant delivery of herbal medicine. Feeling of warmth is soothing itself, and it also helps in reducing muscle spasm when applied. It also helps in vasodilation in specific areas to speed up recovery. Some herbs are delightful in fragrance and thus can provide the body with an unusual odor. Any natural fiber, a cloth with pores or muslin bag, can be used to form compresses from medicinal herbs. In traditional herbal medicine, compresses were formed by putting them in direct sunlight to get the effects of warmth. In modern days, ovens can be used to achieve the temperature and thus applied to the skin in comfortable ways. Microwaving should be avoided when other natural sources are available because of the health hazards of artificial heating. Different and multiple layers are also used over single compress to achieve maximum absorption as well as the mixing of herbs. It also protects from overheating and bruising.

Poultice or Marham is a type of herbal medicine that is applied to skin sores and wounds directly to achieve healing at maximum pace and to unlock bactericidal and anti-inflammatory benefits. It is an excellent source of delivering medicine from the skin to other, more profound layers of the body. Again, it is a popular form of medicine in traditional Chinese, Indian, and Muslim herbalism. It is so easy to apply the poultices that it can be applied to gums in mouth as well as on lips to treat symptoms of herpes and other STDs. Any type of fresh, damp, or dried herbs can be used to make poultices. Another effective way to apply them is to keep them on wounds for more extended periods to achieve maximum absorption. It is a widely used method of administration in herbal dentistry because it is by far the safest method to be used in the oral cavity. A poultice can be left overnight or longer in the mouth to avoid bruising and sores in the mouth. It will also help in improving the freshness of mouth and thus promoting the better odor in breath. It is essential to know the dosage of the herb in a poultice. A poultice is a damp or less wet type of medication, more like a paste which can be made by just mixing water, tea or decoction in a dried paste of herb. A mixture of different herbs can also be used to make a poultice to unlock many benefits hidden in these different herbs. It is a fantastic strategy that is used by many herbalists. For example, an analgesic herb containing pain killer properties can be mixed with antioxidant, anti-inflammatory, or any type of bactericidal herb to achieve all these impacts by a single use of poultice. A great recipe involves the use of herbal tea with blueberry along with willow to unlock the actions of all these three herbs in a single poultice.

The use of herbal medicine in the shape of poultices, washcloths, and compresses provides significant benefits over oral routes when treating skin-related disorders. Our skin is acidic in nature, and skin is the largest organ of the body. Our outlook entirely depends upon our skin, and our diet can clearly be shown by the quality of our skin. Regulation of the skin's pH is obtained through its buffering effects. It helps to normalize the tone and turgor of skin due to its antioxidant nature and by providing the exact nourishment to the surface. Acne is the most frequent skin problem which affects every gender, every age group, and every race of humankind on earth. It is the accumulation of pus that is comprised of dead white blood cells and debris of bacteria killed. Low immunity, increase exposure to infections, and diet reduced in essential components can lead to acne issues. The most typical areas of skin that are prone to acne are facial skin. Herbal medicine very effectively reduces the chances of acne due to its anti-oxidative nature and positive effects on immunity. It also reduces the chances of overproduction of gastric acid, which also causes acne. Moreover, herbal medicine helps in normalizing the pH of our skin, which leads to fewer acne-related episodes. Another benefit of herbal medicine for acne is the reduced production of oil from sebaceous glands of our skin, which is thought to Herbal antivirals the most catastrophic effects related to acne issues. This is the reason that oily skin is most prone to acne-related problems. However, regular use of herbal medicine and diet rich in protein and antioxidants can help us reduce these episodes.

Our skin is much prone to fungal infections. Some colonies of fungus are skin-friendly and usually live on our skin, but some inappropriate exposures of temperature can cause over colonization of this fungus. Tinea versicolor is a similar issue. In this fungal skin infection, skin-friendly and normally living colony of skin fungus get provoked by the exposure of higher temperatures, which leads to the patchy appearance of our skin. Skin becomes multicolored (as the name implies) in this disease. Any treatment which reduces the fungal growth can be useful in this case. Herbal medicine is a potent antifungal. Thermoregulation is one of the most significant impacts of herbal medicine. All these benefits make it a treatment of choice in any kind of fungal skin infections. We will discuss fungal issues of skin in detail later.

Over porous skin and increased freckles are very disturbing for cosmetic purposes. These issues are caused by reduced skin turgor, which can also be age-related. An unbalanced and unhealthy diet also leads to these issues. Herbal medicine helps in maintaining the turgor pressure of our skin as well as helps in detoxifying it. It also helps us regulate our dietary habits, and thus it can provide very superior results in this case. Aging is a process that is natural and universal. It cannot be stopped but can be delayed. Aging reduces the turgor and cosmetic appearance of our skin. It is essential to say that it causes freckles and discoloration of the skin. Aging skin is also more prone to infections and sunburns. Herbal medicine helps in delaying the aging process of skin by providing the right nourishment and balancing the pH of our skin. It also helps in fighting with infection and helps in preserving the natural tone and glow of our skin.

Herbal medicine used as herbal baths:

The largest organ of the body is skin, which has a very complicated structure and very diverse in properties and colors. Skin is porous and can allow transmission of medicine into deep structures when suitable media is used. Teas and decoctions are also used in bathing to enhance the delivery of medicine, for example, in sauna bathing. Hands and feet can be bathed alone in pots filled with herbal water, or full body can be soaked in a bathtub to achieve the medicinal benefits of herbal medicine. In bedridden patients, a damp cloth with medicinal fluid in it is a smart way of medicinal bed bathing. Hot baths are essential because they can make skin porous, and thus more drugs can be administered inside the body. Care should be taken when using a hot water bath to avoid burns and bruising. Bathing can be achieved by directly introducing dried herbs in bathtubs or pots to unlock maximum healing benefits. These herbs can be inserted directly in the bathtub, or these can be introduced in porous clothes like socks, pantyhose, and other delicate clothes to avoid a mess. Even loofa made from herbs can be used to be rubbed on the skin directly to maximize the absorption of the medicine through the skin. It is the smartest way of administration, but it can turn bathtubs a little messy and hard to clean.

Washcloths are indeed a great source to get bathed on the bed. They can be used on a critically ill patient who cannot survive an active bath. In this comfortable way, medicine can easily be applied to the skin, and thus it can be transferred in a deeper area of the body through diffusion. Washcloths can be warm by using hot infusions of medicine when specific impacts of heating are needed, or they can be cold when benefits of cold are needed. It all depends upon personal choice as well as symptoms of illnesses. For acute injuries, for example, brushing and combat sports fights, cold washcloths with specific benefits of ice and anti-inflammatory medicine can be a smart choice to limit swelling and bruising as well as impeding bleeding from fresh wounds. Cold also has anesthetic properties, which make it a natural pain killer. When used warm, washcloths can stimulate blood flow due to vasodilatory effects as well as a soothing response of the body can also be obtained.

Other modes of administrations:

Infants can also use herbal medicine, but the route of administration, as well as dosing, can be very troublesome to decide. A full cup of tea and an ice cube of decoction is a terrible idea when used for infants. We Herbal antivirals to decide the safest routes of administration because of the delicate body of infants. Breast milk is a natural source to nourish babies from the nutrients in the mother's blood. Breast milk is the safest from all the routes of nourishment because many complex nutrients that cannot be introduced in an infant's body otherwise can easily be inserted through breast milk. A mother and her child, both can be benefited in that way. Some herbal medicines are really infant friendly while others can be harsher on the delicate infant body, so a careful consideration before administration is essential to avoid any kind of side effects. Another significant benefit is to insert potent herbal antibacterial medicine inside an infant to make more him/her more immune with side effects of getting sick from antibacterials is to introduce them from the mother's breast milk. It will boost the natural immunization responses in both mother and her infant.

CHAPTER4: HERBAL PLANTS USED IN HERBAL ANTIVIRALS

This chapter with throw light on different characteristics of different herbal medicine used as potent herbal antivirals.

To understand the health benefits of a plant, it is essential to the basic properties of that plant as well as necessary actions of the same plant on different organs and systems of the body. Our body is very complex, and any missing detail can lead to catastrophic effects. The dose of a herb given in specific illnesses should also be very calculated. In this text, we will discuss some fundamental details about nearly each and every plant used in herbalism as a source of herbal medicine.

Acerola

- *Malpighia glabra is the Latin name of this plant*
- This plant comes from Barbados cherry family
- It is fruity in nature.

Details:

This herb is essential because of unusual Vitamin C concentrations and flavin related compounds called flavonoids. It can also have nearly 3900mg of vitamin C, which makes it a perfect choice to boost natural immunity. A little weight of this plant can provide a very high amount of vitamin C so that hypervitaminosis can be a concern. It is also very rich in amazing and effective antioxidants as well as it can also contain a high amount of protein, minerals and salts, iron, and potassium. It also contains calcium and some trace minerals. Another benefit of using acerola as a daily diet is its antifungal actions. It can also be considered as a super fruit. Regular supplementation of this fruit can delays aging and prevention of many deadly and common diseases.

Dosage:

nearly 400-4500mg when used as an extract. In powder form, the required dose is nearly 3-9 grams.

Traditional use:

It is a traditional drink of Brazil, and it is considered as an effective remedy for intestinal issues and frequent fevers. It is also associated with its anti-inflammatory benefits, which can directly affect the liver, heart, and kidneys. It is also used to cure blood-related issues, rheumatic problems, and increased obesity.

Amla or Indian berry:

- *Phyllanthus Emblica* is the Latin name of this plant.
- Amla is an Indian plant, also known as Indian berry.
- It is used as whole fruit, oil extracted, and in powder form.

Details:

It is an artificial plant, as well as a fruit that is berry shaped. The critical factor is the nutritious benefits provided by this fruit, which is rich in very unique and rare benefits. It is an important fruit which can be used in health promotion and anti-aging. It is also called as a super fruit. A vast scientific literature is dedicated to supporting this fruit. It contains high amounts of antioxidants, antifungal, antiviral, disinfectant, and protecting benefits. It is also essential In the reduction of cholesterol from the body and thus reduces the chances of atherosclerosis and heart attacks.

A word Rasayana is used in traditional Indian medicine, which is associated with the global benefits of amla in the human body. Amla is a natural coolant that can be a protective remedy during hot summers. It also has cooling effects on the liver and stomach.

Therapeutic dosing range:

When extracted, amla can be used in 70-1100mg dose.

When in powdered form, the daily dose can be 4-9 grams per day.

Traditional uses:

A word Rasayana is used in traditional Indian medicine, which is associated with the global benefits of amla in the human body. Amla is the natural coolant that can be a protective remedy during hot summers. It also has cooling effects on the liver and stomach.

It is a natural thirst reliever, and thus it is traditionally used in hot climates of India from ancient times. During Indian fasts, which can be forty-day long, amla is used as a protective fruit that can heal the body and protects from getting sick. It is also given to children mixed with sugar to protect them from evil eyes in traditional Indian culture.

Ashwagandha:

- *Withania somnifera* is called in Latin as well as botanically.
- It is also a plant of Indian origin that is widely used for its protective benefits.

Details:

It is a well-known root that is used to relieve pain and other symptoms of joint arthritis, gouty arthritis, stress and anxiety disorder, and sleep disturbances. It is also used to relieve symptoms of asthma and chronic cough. In pregnant females, it is used to relieve issues related to pregnancies, and it is also a natural cure for infertility. Patients with low libido drive and impotence can use this root for sexual benefits.

It is also an essential treatment for aging, and it can cure edema as well as age-related changes in the brain and skin. Its effects on T.B. and other pathogenic disorders, however, need to be established by medical research.

Dosage:

When used in crude quality, 3-9 gram is sufficient.

1-2 ml in fluid form

80-800mg in standard extract

Astragalus

Astragalus membranaceus is the Latin name of this plant. It is of Leguminosae (bean) subclass. It is a widely used plant in China, Japan, and Korea. It is basically a root in morphology

Details:

The importance of this root plant in traditional Chinese herbalism is well known. It is considered a great root to promote the self-healing capacity of the body and to maintain vital forces inside the body.

Some western herbalists also used this root as the primary source of tonic, which is essential to promote natural immunity and vital capacities of the body. This root has some fantastic impacts on neural and endocrinal systems of the body. It can be a primary herbal remedy for patients with deficient immunity or those who are treated by chemotherapy and radiotherapy.

These benefits of the herb make it a herbal remedy of choice for cancer patients all over the world. It is a primary adaptive herbal remedy in oncology. Moreover, the use of astragalus is hazard-free and safe. It has a fantastic impact on bone marrow, and thus, it can easily promote immunity by producing more potent white blood cells that can be used in the war against the deadly pathogens like bacteria and viruses.

The research base of this root for cancer patients is highly relevant to establish its efficacy in the oncology department. It acts on multiple systems of cancer patients and promotes a more safe and healthy lifestyle in cancer patients. This herb is also essential in maintaining health benefits. It has a sweet taste, and it can be used as a powder in cancer patients. The pleasant taste of this herb is essential in more tolerance by cancer patients.

Many recipes associated with this herb promote the use of the herb in the form of smoothies because of its sweet taste and pleasant smell. This fluid form is more consumable for cancer patients. It also helps in improving the digestive health of cardiac patients.

dosage:

10-30 grams when used as a tea or smooth.

If someone wants to make tea, roots slices can be boiled for several minutes, and this technique is derived from traditional Chinese medicine, which also widely practiced in many countries of the world.

When used as a fluid extract, 5-10 ml is sufficient.

Traditional uses:

It has traditional backgrounds for the betterment of vital forces inside a human body. It is a fantastic remedy for weakness, fevers, lack of immunity, deprived focus, aging, and, most importantly, cancer. *Huangqi* is the term which is used as a source of yellow energy, and it is associated with the beneficial use of this herb in Chinese folk medicine. It is named as yellow energy because, in Chinese culture, yellow energy is thought to be associated with the vital forces inside a body which are essential to maintain equilibrium between health and illness. Qi or chi is used as positive energy, and it is thought that this herb is essential in achieving the positive energy in many human organs and systems, especially in the spleen. So, it can be easily understood that the reasons for using this herb in cancer patients are not from a lame theory, but actual uses of this herb against low immunity are clearly shown in the literature.

In China, this root is used as a symbol of defending the energy of the body, and in western medicine, it is synonymous with the word immunity. In traditional Chinese medicine, this root was also used for fever, cough, constipation, diarrhea, vomiting, and flu. It is thought that this herb can be a sufficient insufficient blood flow of the body, and thus, it can be used against peripheral vascular diseases, varicose veins, anemia, and many other blood disorders.

Apple cider vinegar:

During the last decades, medical science has been evolved immensely, and researches are being conducted to find the new and most effective ways of treatments. With the advancement of science, challenges are also growing at a faster rate. Poor lifestyle, increasing weights and body fats, loss of physical activities are causing much distress to the human population. This change of human behavior is causing a shift of healthcare from treatment to prevention, and that is why apple cider vinegar is creating so much hype these days. Apple cider vinegar is not new to medical science, but with the advancement of research and analytics, many unique properties of apple cider vinegar are being studied. It is now proved that apple cider vinegar is a very effective remedy for healthy weight loss, detoxification, and improving overall health.

As the name implies, Apple cider vinegar is produced when cider apples, a bitter and unpalatable type of apples are undergone in fermentation to create vinegar. Cider is an English word, but it got its origin from German and old French culture. It seems very easy, but it is a complicated procedure because there are many steps in producing a high-quality apple cider vinegar. Many different ways are used in its production. Some areas of the world prefer conventional methods, yet the rest of the world is using more advanced and easy to go manufacturing. Many different types of apple cider vinegar are available depending upon the area of production, the type of production, and composition, i.e., stable versus liquid. The distinguishing property between these two types is their taste. Cooker or dessert apple is sweet and more palatable while the cider is bitter and sour. Initially, cider apples were used only for fermentation purposes, while with the advancement of technology, they are also being used for many other purposes.

Classifications of cider apples:

Many classification systems are used for cider apples, but the most crucial classification system is the Long Ashton research station classification system. This system classifies the cider apples into four categories i.e.

Sweets (S.W.): These types are low in tannin and less acidic.

Sharp (S.H.): These are high in tannin levels and more acidic, which makes them eligible to use in apple cider vinegar formation. In Eastern England, these subtypes are being used to make apple cider vinegar.

Bittersweet (BSW): These are the most famous ciders in Europe, and these are also considered as "French" or "Norman" Varieties.

Bittersharp (BSH): these are also considered as "spitters" and have the highest levels of acid and tannin. These are suitable only for fermentation purposes.

Difference between apple juice and apple cider:

Apple cider and apple juice are the products of the same source, i.e., cider apples, but the difference lies in composition. Apple cider is characterized as an unpasteurized and unprocessed liquid. On the other hand, apple juice is the result after heating the apple cider at 190°F, and it is more transparent and processed liquid.

The Mother:

During the conversion process of apple juice into apple cider vinegar, the most critical component is called "the mother." It is a solution rich in cellulose and bacteria's which are friendly and probiotic. Mother solution causes discrimination between processed and unprocessed apple cider vinegar. Unprocessed apple cider vinegar has more mother solution leftovers and vice versa. It is thought that it is the mother who gives the apple cider vinegar its nutritional benefits, and that is the reason raw and unprocessed apple cider vinegar is superior to processed one.

Formation of apple cider vinegar:

Apple cider vinegar can be homemade or commercially produced. It can be processed or unprocessed. It all depends upon the primary solution, "the mother."

Apple cider vinegar is produced in the following ways:

Extraction:

In this step, cider apples are crushed, and juice is extracted from them.

First fermentation:

In this step, apple juice is mixed with mother, a solution that is rich in cellulose and probiotic bacteria and yeast. This step converts the sugars into alcohol.

Second fermentation:

In this step, the alcohol is transformed into vinegar by acetobacter, i.e., bacteria which produce acid. The reasons behind the bitter and sour taste of apple cider are the malic and acetic acid.

Types of apple cider vinegar:

Apple cider vinegar can be classified based on production, type, origin, and composition.

Classification based upon production:

Homemade apple cider vinegar:

Cider apples are cut into cubes to increase the exposed area, which helps the bacteria to work. A is made by mixing water and sugars. Honey can be used as an alternative to sugars. Apple cubes are submerged in the solution and kept for almost two weeks in any pot with breathable cover on it. Then it is strained and held for nearly four more weeks to get the desired product, i.e., apple cider vinegar.

Commercial apple cider vinegar:

Machines and belts are used for crushing the cider apples in industrial plants. Then they are squeezed to extract the juice. In a tank, the solution is exposed to oxygen, and this storage turns the liquid into alcohol when it is strained with acetobacter (first fermentation). In the second fermentation, alcohol is deformed into acetic acid and malic acid, which turns it into vinegar. In most commercial plants, apple cider vinegar is pasteurized, leaving no trace of the mother, and thus, a bright, less smelly fluid is obtained.

Classification based upon types:

Cider can be classified as processed and unprocessed. These are also called regular and raw apple cider vinegar, respectively. In both examples, cider apples are used to produce apple cider vinegar, and the difference lies in the result.

Unprocessed apple cider vinegar:

Unprocessed apple cider vinegar is not pasteurized and contains the mother, a component used in the formation of apple cider vinegar. This is a raw liquid with a cloudy appearance, and it has a typical smell of apples.

Processed apple cider vinegar:

Processed or regular apple cider vinegar is the type which we get after boiling the apple cider vinegar at 190°F, a process called pasteurization. That turns the end product into a bright and less smelly liquid.

Classification based upon origin:

English apple cider vinegar:

In this type, sharp cider apples that are classified by the Long Ashton research station classification system are used. It is most common in Eastern England.

French/European apple cider vinegar:

Bittersweet (BSW) type cider apples are used in this type according to the Long Ashton research station classification system. It is most common in European and American areas.

Classification based upon composition:

Liquid:

It is the most common type available

Solid:

Some manufacturers of modern days are also providing apple cider vinegar in the solid form, e.g., in the form of tablets and gums.

Properties of apple cider vinegar:

Chemical properties:

Apple cider vinegar contains an abundant amount of acetic and melic acid, which makes it alkaline, and its pH is about 2-3.

Biotic properties:

Apple cider vinegar contains useful bacteria called probiotic bacteria, which are highly effective in reducing stomach acid, improve digestion, and boost immunity.

Nutritional properties:

potassium. This element is used by our bodies to perform multiple functions, e.g., to maintain heart rate and increasing efficiency of skeletal muscle. It contains acetic and melic acid, which improve digestion and effectively kill dangerous bacteria because they cannot sustain an acidic medium. Moreover, raw apple cider vinegar contains enzymes, catalysts, amino acids, fiber, and suitable lipids, which are very useful in many ways.

Healing properties:

Skin is acidic, and apple cider vinegar causes wonders in improving the skin by rebalancing its pH. It heals the inner layer of our stomach, which protects the stomach from gastric acid. Enzymes and catalysts in raw apple cider vinegar are essential in boosting wound healing after injury. Some trials have shown its effectiveness in healing the scalp and hairs.

Antibacterial properties:

The list of apple cider vinegar uses very long, and it has been proven an effective treatment of many illnesses since ancient times. Essential benefits of apple cider vinegar are:

Catalyst properties:

Apple cider vinegar acts as a catalyst in the breakdown of food into macro and micronutrients. Vinegar is being used since ancient times for the softening of meat and making it more edible and digestible.

Uses:

The list of herbal antivirals uses very long, and it has been proven an effective treatment of many illnesses since ancient times. Essential benefits of herbal antivirals are:

Potent Antibacterial:

Apple cider vinegar is a potent antibacterial substance that can protect us against many dangerous bacteria. Bacteria contain a lipid coating that is vulnerable to the acidic environment. Acetic acid and overall alkaline pH of apple cider vinegar make it highly unsuitable for these dangerous bacteria. The friendly bacteria present in apple cider vinegar promote the colonies of E.coli, which are present in our intestines and improve digestion.

Vitamin C is a vitamin of immunity. Apple cider vinegar is very rich in vitamin C and thus has a direct impact on our resistance. Because of higher vitamin C concentrations, apple cider vinegar is the best source to boost our immunity and thus to improve overall health. Our body is always under some inflammatory process because healing and the damaging cycle is still on the go. In inflammation, free oxygen radicals are produced, and the intensity of inflammation is characterized by the frequency of production of reactive oxygen species. Apple cider vinegar guards our bodies against inflammatory processes by reducing the reactive oxygen species.

Bilberry

- *Vaccinium myrtillus* is the Latin name of the plant.
- It belongs to the health family botanically.
- Another name of the plant is wild blueberry.
- Both leaves and berries of the plant are used in herbal medicine. Uva ursi is the name implies to the leaves of this plant, which Is used for the treatment of UTIs (urinary tract infection).

Details:

This plant belongs to the Ericaceae family, and the common name implies to this plant is a blueberry plant. It has proven benefits for eye health, and ocular pathologies can easily be treated by its herbal use. It is essential to the aging process in the eyes and to improve night vision. Cataract and ocular degeneration can be controlled by its regular use. Eye weakness and blindness affect a considerable population in the world, and using the blueberry can prevent these issues.

Dosage:

500mg of pure extract is sufficient together with all the benefits provided by this plant. If it is used in capsular form, 1-3 capsules daily can be a smart idea.

Traditional uses:

For many centuries, blueberry is the fruit of choice in western culture to make pies and cakes. Sweet dishes Herbal antivirals an essential part of blueberries in western culture. It also has a great medicinal history in traditional western and Chinese culture. As an artist of the western era, Hildegard has allegedly used blueberries in his mystic music as a source of menses in females. Historically, blueberries were used to treat frequent cough and fever, kidney stones, intestinal bloating, liver disorders, piles, and infections of the dermis and oral mucosa. Many American herbalists of ancient times used blueberries against diabetes. It was thought of as a potent source of insulin. The use of blueberries in ocular issues is widespread. It has proven benefits for eye health, and ocular pathologies can easily be treated by its herbal use. It is essential to delay the aging process in the eyes and to improve night vision. Cataract and ocular degeneration can be controlled by its regular use. Eye weakness and blindness affect a considerable population in the world, and using the blueberry can prevent these issues.

An essential historical debate about blueberries is the use of this plant in world war 2. It was a very famous plant among the pilots of the Air force. Jam made of blueberries was used before the night attacks to prevent night blindness. Glaucoma and diabetic eye diseases were also treated by regular uses of blueberries. In Europe, surgeons used blueberries for the quick healing of wounds. Brushing, hemorrhoids, and piles are treated in herbalism by using blueberry pastes. The use of blueberries to treat diarrhea is also a debate of great importance. The fibrous nature of this fruit is essential to relieve constipation, which is the hardening of stool, and nearly every human and of every age suffer from this disorder many times in his/her life. All these historical, as well as modern times benefits, are enough to consider blueberries as a super fruit. However, the use of blueberries in Indian traditional culture is not very common because these re tough to grow in that habitat.

Devil's Club

- *Oplopanax horridus* is the Latin word of this herb.
- This plant belongs to the ginseng family, and botanically, it is considered in the Araliaceae family. Another name implied to this plant is Devil's stick or Devil's walking cane. Its roots leave as well as stem are used for herbal medicinal purposes in herbalism.
- It should not be confused with the devil's claw, which is a plant grown in hot deserts.

Details:

This plant is widely produced in the northwest of America. It also contains many attributes of the ginseng family, which is essential to treat diabetes. It helps in curing the insulin resistance. It also helps in lowering the increased cholesterol levels in the blood. The most significant benefit of this herb is its use in weight loss and weight management coach, who knows its herbal impact can help his/her client to reduce some extra pounds in a natural and effective manner. This plant is really a blessing for diabetic patients because it helps in increasing the blood insulin levels and reducing the blood glucose spike after meals, which can be dangerous for pre-diabetics and full-blown diabetic patients. Its anti-inflammatory and antioxidant nature helps in recovery if cancer patients because it helps in reducing the weight and extra fat in cancer patients, which is caused due to stress. Cancer patients also possess poor insulin tolerance, and thus, it helps in this regard as well.

Dosage:

When it is used in fluid form. 2-5 ml consumption of this syrup for 2-3 times a day can be a smart idea.

Traditional uses:

It is a much-used herb in Alaska and Great Britain. It was also widely used in the folk medicine of Columbia. The most prominent benefits of using this herb are to use it against joint and gouty arthritis, common fever and cough, and against diabetes. The use of this plant against diabetes is highly prominent. Natives of Alaska were found to use a herbal drink of this plant to cure cancer. They also used it for weight reduction and lowering extra pounds from the body. The use of this plant in Alaskan natives for constipation, diarrhea, stomach and skin ulcers as well as gallstones are many folds. In some traditional and folk medicine, this herb was used to increase sexuality and libido among men, and it was also used to increase menstruation in females. It was also used to restore the proper menstruation cycle after birth. The stem, leaves, and branches of this herb were used to treat the focus, attentional and mental health among society.

Ginger:

- *Zingiber officinale* is the official botanic name of this herb.
- It belongs to Zingiberaceae family botanically
- The most used part of this plant in the world is its root.

Details:

It is a well-known root which is used widely in every corner and every country in the world. It is used because of its millions of benefits which need no special consideration. Research background about this herb is highly sufficient to prove its benefits in the area of healthcare and medicine.

It is a Universal herbal agent. It is known as a cooking spice in most areas of the world. Moreover, its herbal uses in medicine and healthcare are not hidden, and it is one of the most used herbal medicine agents around the globe.

It is a world's well-known herbal spice and most favorite remedy to treat infections and inflammations. Many homemakers and mothers from the historical point of view used this herb to treat the most common illnesses of daily households. The most significant benefits associated with this herb are fever, pain associated with burns and injuries, and flu. It is also widely used for common colds and Asian flu. One of the most important benefits of ginger is on the mesentery. The human intestine is a loopy structure, and it is subjected to many illnesses due to food and infections. Bowel gas affects nearly every human being on earth, and every age is prone to this illness. Human bowel gases can cause abdominal distention and stress. Ginger is a historically proven remedy for gaseous issues. It is essential to maintain the primary media of intestine so that fewer infections can affect it, and it is also essential to increase the abdominal sufficiency related to the digestion and excretion of food.

Another significant benefit of ginger is its effects on respiration and common colds. Mostly in children, frequent colds and flu affect health due to common influenza viruses which involve millions of human beings around the globe every year. Ginger is essential to shield against these common influenza infections. It is also essential in clearing the breathing tracts from mouth to lungs, and thus it helps in preventing the symptoms of asthma and choking. It also helps in clearing the mucous from respiratory tracts. Another benefit of ginger is removing the foul odor of breathing. It prevents, treats, or shortens the symptoms of respiratory illnesses.

Another benefit of ginger is on indigestion and proper production of gastric juice. Gastric juice is essential to digest the food, and it helps in softening the food, which will then pass to the small and large intestines. Ginger helps in producing stomach acids in sufficient quantities to help indigestion. Gastric juice, when overproduced, can cause much sore breaths, stomachaches, and irritation. It is essential to regulate the proper concentrations of stomach acid to avoid any disturbances. Ginger is an extraordinary remedy to reduce the overproduction of gastric acid as well as increasing the underproduced amounts of gastric acid to improve the digestion issues.

The human intestine is loopy structures and extensive tracts to digest and finally excrete the food. Infection-related to the intestine can cause symptoms of diarrhea and constipation, as well as bloating and abdominal pains. Ginger helps in regulating the media of intestine, and thus it helps in improving intestinal health and helps in preventing the symptoms of diarrhea and constipation. Interestingly ginger also helps in reducing the inflammation of the intestine, which is associated with irritable bowel syndrome and many other inflammatory diseases of the abdomen.

It is a potent antioxidant herb that is essential in regulating the anti-inflammatory pathways of the body. Ginger helps in reducing the free oxygen radicals and highly reactive oxygen species, which can cause issues related to cell injury and cytotoxicity. It helps in detoxification of skin to make it more glowing and beautiful. It helps in reducing the redness and inflammation in eyes so that it makes them brighter and shiny as well. Ginger also helps in regulating the hormones of the body. So it is an important herb that is used in traditional Chinese medicine, Indian ayurvedic medicine as well as modern western medicine to treat the symptoms of impotence and low libido drive. It is a primary male aphrodisiac agent who is also associated with increase blood levels of testosterone as well as increased healthy sperms in semen.

Another essential benefit of ginger is the inhibition of thromboxane, which is essential in gathering and clotting from platelets. Thus inhibition of platelet is essential to reduce the inflammation in the body. This characteristic makes ginger a vital herb to reduce the signs of fever and common colds. Unlike other herbs already discussed in this chapter, ginger is a potent stimulating agent fr diaphoresis. This benefit makes it an excellent remedy to improve the blood flow in peripheral vessels as well as reducing the chances of blood clotting and deep venous thrombosis, which is a common problem in patients who are overweight and bedridden. It is also essential in regulating the heartrates in the body. It is a potent thermogenic herb that increases the temperature of the body and thus increases the overall metabolism of the body as well. It is an important herb to decrease the cholesterol levels from blood because of its lipolytic actions and a strong affinity with fats, which helps to excrete them from the body. It helps in increasing the saliva and production of bile from the gall bladder to increase the digestion of fats from the body and the reduction of free fatty acids from the blood. It is also an essential herb to prevent vomiting and morning sickness in pregnant females and chronically ill patients. It is an important herb to reduce the signs of osteoarthritis, rheumatoid arthritis, and gouty arthritis because of its benefits against the inflammatory mediators of the body.

The therapeutic benefits of ginger are millions, and a complete text can be dedicated to considering the details of these benefits. However, this book is a short guide for beginners abut herbalism, and all these mind-blowing benefits cannot be covered here in detail.

From a herbalist point of view, ginger can be considered as the most crucial herb of the history because its use is from millions of years as well as, nearly every civilization has used this herb to gather some astounding benefits from it. Details will be covered in traditional use sections.

To conclude the benefits of ginger, it is essential to say that t can be used in every type of illness and pathology with fear of side effects or adverse reactions to the body because it is one of the most human-friendly types of herb ever known historically.

Dosing:

1-2 grams of a dried form of this herb two to three times per day is an effective strategy to unlock millions of benefits associated with this herb.

When used in the form of fluid extract, the same 1-2ml of fluid is sufficient to help reduce many illnesses when used three times daily.

When used in powdered form, 100 to 400 mg of powder twice or thrice daily can be an essential bet to make.

Some herbalists also use the super extract of this herb in 40 to 80mg concentration two to three times per day to achieve maximum benefits.

Traditional uses:

It is known that ginger was used for more than 2000 years in traditional Chinese medicine to treat nausea and vomiting related symptoms. It was also used in Chinese medicine to cure bleeding diseases because of platelet dysfunctions in the body as well in the treatment of rheumatic and gouty arthritis. Another use of ginger in traditional Chinese medicine was to treat the symptoms of snakebite and other venomous stinks. It was also a very potent herb used in the treatment of pain in gums and teeth. Stomach and intestine related issues were also treated by using this herb in traditional Chinese medicine. It is also used as an excellent remedy to treat intestinal gases and abdominal distentions. Ginger was considered as a shield against hard winters because it was an extraordinary remedy to treat the symptoms of frostbite due to its thermogenic properties. These thermogenic properties of this herb were also fundamental to treat the symptoms of cold extremities, weak and bounding pulse, cough, and fever as well as flu. Traditional Chinese medicine also used this herb in summers and damp weather.

In India, Ayurveda used this herb to prevent cardiac arrest due to blood clotting and to fight against the symptoms of atherosclerosis in the arteries of the heart. In Malaysia and other Asian countries, soups rich in ginger were given to the new mothers after delivering their babies to increase sweating and perforations so that impurities can be excreted from the body after birth. In Arabic and traditional Muslim medicine, ginger was used to increase the maleness and testosterone. In traditional African medicine, ginger is used to treat the symptoms as a mosquito repellent herb. Western traditional herbalism used this herb in the form of infusion to treat congestion and pain associated with the female menstrual cycle. Ginger has the potency to decrease pain and abdominal cramps in menstruating females. Ginger was used In nearly every culture, and it was used for nearly every type of illness of humankind due to its great health benefits. In some herbalism cultures, ginger was also used as a flavoring and fragrant agent to build different types of scents and perfumes with hundreds of therapeutic benefits. In short, ginger is a complete type of super herb in human history.

CHAPTER5: RECIPES FOR HOMEMADE HERBAL ANTIVIRALS; A MULTIPURPOSE GUIDE:

Herbal medicine can be made at home in the form of teas, tinctures, washcloths, and oils. Some forms also use external ways of application, for example, baths.

Now, we will discuss a different way of herbal medicine preparation and administration at home:

Teas:

Tea is well known and probably the most consumed beverage in the world. The use of this herb for medicinal purposes is well known and has a strong research background. Black tea requires the essential and partial fermentation process of the tea leaves. However, green tea doesn't require these kinds of fermentation and can be produced through the process of steaming the leaves. This process reduces the oxidation capacities of enzymes present in tea leaves, and the preservation of polyphenol is achieved through this process. It is interesting to know that Polyphenols belong to a family of flavonoids which are present 30-40 percent of the total weight in dried green tea leaves. Camellia sinensis is a known name of dried and unfermented green tea leaves. It has a property to reduce bacterial and viral activities in the body. It is also essential in lowering down the increased concentration of lipids in the blood. The potency of green tea to lower down the blood cholesterol level is excellent, and thus it is a beverage of choice to reduce some extra pounds from the body. It is a potent anti-lipidemic agent. Its antioxidant benefits make it a perfect choice to detoxify the liver, kidneys, intestine, stomach, and skin. Its detoxifying and lipid-lowering benefits make it a perfect choice as a natural healer. The scientific base behind green tea is solid, and it is used in traditional as well as modern medicine as a natural source to treat many common illnesses of the human body. It is a super herb in holism, and the benefits of this herb are beyond the capacity of this essential book on holism.

Dosing of tea depends upon different factors and situations. When used in acute disorders and illnesses, the current complaint guides the dosage. Acute conditions may require multiple doses per day as compared to chronic doses, which require fewer doses for a prolonged time. Herbal medicine incorporates dosage according to the individual needs of a person rather than just treating symptoms with predetermined dosing strategies. It is not essential to stick with a specific pattern of dosing, and it can vary according to personal needs and interests, which is not practice when it comes to western allopathic medicine.

Teas are made from the specific plants of the tea family, and leaves of tea plants are mostly used in this process. However, other parts, such as flowers, can also be used. It can be made from dried or fresh parts of tea making plants, and the servings per day can vary from 2-6 doses depending upon personal needs and tolerance. Sampling mixing the leaves of tea plants in a hot water cup and mixing with honey can provide thousands of health benefits, or it can be made by proper boiling and adding milk, etc. which is called actual fermentation of tea such as black tea.

Tea can be made from handpicked leaves of tea plant grown in self botanic gardens, or it can be made from pre-designed herbal tea bags for convenience. When aromatic tea sources such as rosemary are used, its steam can also provide a face freshening treatment, which is a common practice in many western and Indian ayurvedic beauty treatments. Artificial or natural sweeteners such as honey can be used for adding more flavor to herbal teas. Stevia teas are naturally lovely in taste. Take a pinch of stevia tea, cool it in open-air then put it in a freezer bag. Then these bags can be put flat in freezers. When hit, a layer of frozen stevia tea can be break into ice chips, which can be used in other drinks to sweeten them as well as many benefits of stevia tea can be obtained through this process in regular drinks.

Decoctions

Decoctions are widely used sources of herbal medicine in herbalism. When roots or barks of plants contain medicinal benefits, it is hard to obtain extracts from these hard parts of plants, such as willow bark. Decoctions are great ways when the extraction of herbal medicine is required from these hard parts of plants. To obtain this, simmer the herb in hot water pan for at least twelve to thirty minutes on low flame. 1:32 ratio is essential to obtain decoctions from the herbs. A commonly used recipe involves 30 grams of herb and 1000ml of water.

Teas and decoctions are widely used as a herbal source of medicine preparation, and the reason behind using them on a wide-scale is easy to use properties. Just sipping through the cup is all it requires to administer the medicine inside the body. Even rinses and gargles can also be made from these two sources to relieve symptoms related to mouth and throat diseases.

Uses in the kitchen:

Herbal antivirals are made in the kitchen and help in saving our kitchen from fungus, molds, damping, and bad odor. It helps to disinfect the dishes and increases the taste of our food. It can also help us in removing the stains of grease and oil from our burner and exhaust.

Recipe: Add two tablespoon of herbal antivirals in 2 cups of water, and one tablespoon of lemon juice can also be added. Keep this fluid inside a porous jar, and this can be kept inside the kitchen for pleasant odor and disinfection. Add two tablespoons of vinegar in regular dishwashing fluid, and it will do miracles to your dishes. It is a potent disinfecting solution which will help you in the prevention of many deadly infections. By spraying the herbal antivirals and lemon juice solution on grease and oil stains, you can be surprised the immediate removal of these stubborn stains. Kitchen draws are more prone to damping, and thus it increases the chances of fungal growth inside your kitchen cabinets. Spray a solution of herbal antivirals, lemon juice, and baking soda on these spaces, and it will suck up all the moisture.

Uses in cleaning:

Our floors are full of germs, and a powerful cleaning solution is always a good idea to fight against bacteria and viruses. Herbal antivirals can do miracles to your clean hygiene. By using herbal antivirals, you can clean your bathroom, toilets, kitchen, halls, gadgets, and nearly everything in your house. It is a potent disinfectant, and the organic nature of herbal antivirals reduces its side effects too much extent. So it will be a wise decision if you make your cleaning solution instead of relying on chemical-based brands.

Recipe: add four tablespoon herbal antivirals, two tablespoon lemon juice, baking soda, 30ml rubbing alcohol in one bucket of water. Mop the floor and tiles. Put the solution in a spray bottle cloth as per your desire. This highly disinfectant solution can also be added to your regular cleaning fluid.

Uses in the laundry:

Our clothes contain so many germs that we can never imagine. Our garments are our social gadgets. We use them in every event of our life. Chances of contamination of our garments are much higher than any other thing. It is hard to disinfect our clothes than cleaning our body parts. However, by adding herbal antivirals, we can achieve this goal very quickly. That will not only clean our clothes, but it will also provide a pleasant smell to them.

Recipe: add two tablespoons of raw, undiluted herbal antivirals in a washing machine full of warm water. Let the solution get absorbed and then add clothes to the device. Add your regular detergent, and the job is done. You can mix one or two tbsp of herbal antivirals in 2 cups of water, and one tablespoon of lemon juice can also be added. Keep this fluid inside a porous jar, and this can be kept inside the cloth cabinet for pleasant odor and disinfection.

Uses in massage:

Everyone loves a pleasing massage experience, but we should be careful about infections. Our bodies are exposed to germs during the massage. Natural massage oils are not disinfectant in nature, and they can even act as a reservoir of bacteria and fungi. Adding herbal antivirals in your regular massage oil will do wonders.

Recipe: Add a sufficient amount of herbal antivirals in your massage oil. You can also add lemon juice for added detoxification. You can also use only herbal antivirals as a disinfectant bath, but be careful about sensitive areas like eyes, genitals, and open wounds.

Uses in deodorants:

The pleasant smell of herbal antivirals makes it a natural and organic deodorant that has added safety and addition disinfectant and antioxidant characteristics. So, it will be a wise decision to prefer herbal antivirals over chemically prepared deodorants in the market.

Recipe: The recipe to make homemade and natural deodorant is quite easy. Just take a sufficient amount of herbal antivirals in hand apply it on your underarms. You can also use it as a potent aftershave solution because of its disinfecting nature. Herbal antivirals also help in removing the smell of sweat and perspiration. You can add herbal antivirals, lemon juice, and water along with essential oil of your choice inside a spray bottle and keep it with you. By spraying it on your face, hands, and neck every 20 minutes will give you a pleasant and refreshing experience. It is a natural hand sanitizer.

Uses as an air freshener:

You can use herbal antivirals as a natural air freshener for your house or office, and it is no tricky at all.

Recipe: You can use one or two tbsp of herbal antivirals into your regular fluid-based air freshener and use it. You can also make deodorant sticks socked in herbal antivirals, which can be used as a natural air freshener.

Popsicles:
Popsicle is most famous among children and adults as a source of sweet taste, and it is an excellent source of reducing inflammation

and pain related to the oral mucosa. Another benefit of popsicle is its incredible taste and ease of use.

Ice cubes

Ice cubes are a fantastic source of herbal delivery, and they are straightforward to administer. It can be made from teas and decoctions as well. Liquid herbal medicine can be frozen after boiling and rapid cooling, a process called thawing. It also contains pain-relieving benefits, which are very specific with cold therapy. If we add sticks inside ice cubes, they can easily be turned into homemade sweet popsicles. This form of administration is highly famous among children. The ice bags and trays should be labeled accordingly to avoid issues.

Wash clothes:

Washcloths are indeed a great source to get bathed on the bed. They can be used on a critically ill patient who cannot survive an active bath. In this comfortable way, medicine can easily be applied to the skin, and thus it can be transferred in a deeper area of the body through diffusion. Washcloths can be warm by using hot infusions of medicine when specific impacts of heating are needed, or they can be cold when benefits of cold are needed. It all depends upon personal choice as well as symptoms of illnesses. For acute injuries, for example, brushing and combat sports fights, cold washcloths with specific benefits of ice and anti-inflammatory medicine can be a smart choice to limit swelling and bruising as well as impeding bleeding from fresh wounds. Cold also has anesthetic properties, which make it a natural pain killer.

When used warm, washcloths can stimulate blood flow due to vasodilatory effects as well as a soothing response of the body can also be obtained.

Compresses:

Compresses are warm medicinal pastes which are formed from many potent herbs. It is a very traditional technique, which is also caller "Marham" in Arabic, and it is the most used technique in Indian ayurvedic as well. Warm herbs in the form of compresses can stay longer than washcloths on the skin and can be a great source of constant delivery of herbal medicine. Feeling of warmth is soothing itself, and it also helps in reducing muscle spasm when applied. It also helps in vasodilation in specific areas to speed up recovery. Some herbs are delightful in fragrance and thus can provide the body with an unusual odor. Any natural fiber, a cloth with pores or muslin bag, can be used to form compresses from medicinal herbs. In traditional herbal medicine, compresses were formed by putting them in direct sunlight to get the effects of warmth. In modern days, ovens can be used to achieve the temperature and thus applied to the skin in comfortable ways. Microwaving should be avoided when other natural sources are available because of the health hazards of artificial heating. Different and multiple layers are also used over single compress to achieve maximum absorption as well as the mixing of herbs. It also protects from overheating and bruising.

Poultices:

Poultice or Marham is a type of herbal medicine that is applied to skin sores and wounds directly to achieve healing at maximum pace and to unlock bactericidal and anti-inflammatory benefits. It is an excellent source of delivering medicine from the skin to other, more profound layers of the body. Again, it is a popular form of medicine in traditional Chinese, Indian, and Muslim herbalism. It is so easy to apply the poultices that it can be applied to gums in mouth as well as on lips to treat symptoms of herpes and other STDs. Any type of fresh, damp, or dried herbs can be used to make poultices. Another effective way to apply them is to keep them on wounds for more extended periods to achieve maximum absorption. It is a widely used method of administration in herbal dentistry because it is by far the safest method to be used in the oral cavity. A poultice can be left overnight or longer in the mouth to avoid bruising and sores in the mouth. It will also help in improving the freshness of mouth and thus promoting the better odor in breath. It is essential to know the dosage of the herb in a poultice. A poultice is a damp or less wet type of medication, more like a paste which can be made by just mixing water, tea or decoction in a dried paste of herb. A mixture of different herbs can also be used to make a poultice to unlock many benefits hidden in these different herbs. It is a fantastic strategy that is used by many herbalists. For example, an analgesic herb containing pain killer properties can be mixed with antioxidant, anti-inflammatory, or any type of bactericidal herb to achieve all these impacts by a single use of poultice. A great recipe involves the use of herbal tea with blueberry along with willow to unlock the actions of all these three herbs in a single poultice.

Tinctures

Tinctures are drops of herbs in liquid form, which are combined in 80-95% of the alcohol base. The most crucial benefit of this type of administration is the very long preservation period of medicine achieved by adding alcohol into it. It is such a diluted form of medicine that hardly any side effect can occur. This is the sole reason that homeopaths used these types of tinctures from centuries to administer drugs in human bodies. The tincture can be prepared by mixing herb into wine, vodka, or rum. A more diluted media such as herbal antivirals or glycerine can also be used to achieve these benefits. Alcohol-free media can also be used to make tinctures of very diluted quality for those who don't like alcohol to get ingested. Tinctures can be prepared in homes as well as they can also be available in markets. However, the best practice is to make it at home because it doesn't require any special treatment to prepare all these effective tinctures at home. Lany herbalists are famous for making their own tinctures. Raw alcohol is best to make tinctures rather than flavored vodka or rum so that the maximum benefits of herbs can be preserved. Flavoring is also rich in dirty surfers, which are not the right choice for medicinal purposes. Grain alcohol is the most popular type of alcohol used by herbalists to achieve the preparation of the highest quality tinctures. Vodka and grain are very different because they are made from very different sources. Twenty percent net alcohol should be used when the dried herb is made, and 40% of alcohol can be mixed with the fresh herb to ensure proper mixture and administration without side effects.

Willow bark is known to Herbal antivirals high tannin concentration, and thus adding a few amounts of glycerin can be a smart idea for extracting maximum concentration of herb. A tincture is nothing when inferior ingredients are used. Alcohol is just a base in it; however, the medicinal benefits of a tincture can only be achieved from using proper herbs only. A perfect ratio is 1:5, that is 1 part alcohol with five parts of herbs to ensure more concentration of herb in a tincture. This guide is a critical ad accepted in herbalist society all over the world.

. In the case of yarrow, we make an alcohol-based. Yarrow or other types of tannin-containing herbs can be mixed with glycerine and alcohol to extract the medicinal benefits from them properly. The next stage is to put the solution in a dark room while keeping the solution in a tight jar for more than three weeks. A proper shaking the jar every week can also promote proper extraction of the herbal medicinal benefits.

The use of tea and decoction, along with water, can also be applied while making an alcohol free tincture. The final step of tincturing is to stain the solution. The solution is called menstruum, which, while stained, is called a tincture. It is essential to label the jar with the proper name for identification purposes.

These are common and most effective techniques to prepare proper herbal medications at home with much effort and preparation.

Herbal antivirals have multiple uses in the bath, massage, deodorant, home disinfection, dishwashing, cloth washing, disinfecting of toilets, mold and fungus treatment, damp reduction, and air freshening. We will discuss every aspect of herbal antivirals related to these topics in this chapter.

Uses in bath:

Herbal antivirals can help in a pleasant bathing experience. We mostly encounter with hard and contaminated water during bathing, which can be dangerous. Moreover, our bathtubs and showers are contaminated with fungi and algae. These can be very allergic in nature and can also cause plantar warts and fungal infections. So a hygienic bath routine is essential for complete health. Herbal antivirals, through its antifungal capacity, help in the reduction of fungus and algae from our bath place as well as from our body. The antioxidant nature of herbal antivirals helps in reducing the harmful ions, and radicles from our body, which leads to a better and glowing skin condition. Herbal antivirals help in maintaining the pH of the water so that harmful effects and heavy and acidic water are reduced by using herbal antivirals. Another benefit of herbal antivirals is a pleasant odor, which is provided by the herbal antivirals to our body and bath place. This keeps us fresh, healthy, and confidant all day long.

The largest organ of the body is skin, which has a very complicated structure and very diverse in properties and colors. Skin is porous and can allow transmission of medicine into deep structures when suitable media is used. Teas and decoctions are also used in bathing to enhance the delivery of medicine, for example, in sauna bathing. Hands and feet can be bathed alone in pots filled with herbal water, or full body can be soaked in a bathtub to achieve the medicinal benefits of herbal medicine. In bedridden patients, a damp cloth with medicinal fluid in it is a smart way of medicinal bed bathing. Hot baths are essential because they can make skin porous, and thus more drugs can be administered inside the body. Care should be taken when using a hot water bath to avoid burns and bruising. Bathing can be achieved by directly introducing dried herbs in bathtubs or pots to unlock maximum healing benefits. These herbs can be inserted directly in the bathtub, or these can be introduced in porous clothes like socks, pantyhose, and other delicate clothes to avoid a mess. Even loofa made from herbs can be used to be rubbed on the skin directly to maximize the absorption of the medicine through the skin. It is the smartest way of administration, but it can turn bathtubs a little messy and hard to clean.

Recipe: Add two tablespoon of herbal antivirals in 2 cups of water, and one tablespoon of lemon juice can also be added. Keep this fluid inside a porous jar, and this can be kept inside the bathroom for pleasant odor and disinfection. You can also add 1-2 cups of herbal antivirals in the bathtub, which can provide a complete disinfectant and antioxidant bathing experience. The application of apple cider on the face and body frequently as possible by keeping it inside a spray bottle. You can also add essential oils to the solution for a more pleasant experience.

Breast milk:

Infants can also use herbal medicine, but the route of administration, as well as dosing, can be very troublesome to decide. A full cup of tea and an ice cube of decoction is a terrible idea when used for infants. We Herbal antivirals to decide the safest routes of administration because of the delicate body of infants. Breast milk is a natural source to nourish babies from the nutrients in the mother's blood. Breast milk is the safest from all the routes of nourishment because many complex nutrients that cannot be introduced in an infant's body otherwise can easily be inserted through breast milk. A mother and her child, both can be benefited in that way. Some herbal medicines are really infant friendly while others can be harsher on the delicate infant body, so a careful consideration before administration is essential to avoid any kind of side effects. Another significant benefit is to insert potent herbal antibacterial medicine inside an infant to make more him/her more immune with side effects of getting sick from antibacterials is to introduce them from the mother's breast milk. It will boost the natural immunization responses in both mother and her infant.

CHAPTER6: MODE OF ACTIONS OF HERBAL ANTIVIRALS ON VITAL ORGANS

Effects on brain health:

Anatomy: Brain is a soft organ present within the skull and submerged in a fluid called cerebrospinal fluid. The transportation of material is possible through the blood-brain barrier as blood cannot enter the brain directly. The brain is nearly a size of a medium apple, and grooves and ridges are present throughout its morphology.

Physiology: Brain acts as a transformer to control the overall actions of our body. You can consider it as a grid system in which currents Herbal antivirals been passing all the time. It sends and receives signals to and from the spinal cord, interpret it with the relevant memory, and commands relevant actions.

Benefits of HERBAL ANTIVIRALS: herbal antivirals has many direct and indirect benefits over brain health. Directly, it improves the functional capacity of the brain by detoxification of brain media. This action is still understudied. Indirectly, herbal antivirals improve brain function by promoting the absorption of useful substances through the blood-brain barrier by its catalytic properties. It also reduces the chances of deep venous thrombosis and prevents atherosclerosis (plaque formation in blood vessels), and these two conditions can lead to dislodging of thrombi. These thrombi (fat plagues) when dislodged are called emboli. If these emboli enter the brain, they can cause acute disruption of blood supply and can lead to stroke and, ultimately, death. By reducing the chances of plaque and thrombus formation via its lipolytic and anti-cholesterol properties, herbal antivirals indirectly protect the brain. Another essential benefit of herbal antivirals is the improvement of memory. Researches showed that our memory is prone to deteriorate as an aging process, but a junk diet and an unhealthy lifestyle can promote dementia and related pathologies. By improving overall health and through its antioxidant properties, herbal antivirals can reduce the chances of dementia, Parkinsonism, and much other related pathology. Fatigue is another crucial aspect to be discussed here. Mental fatigue is related to the exhausting of the brain after prolonged functioning or reduced brain capacities, which can lead to general body pains and low self-esteem. By providing the nutritional supply to the brain, herbal antivirals can help to prevent the mental as well as general fatigue.

Effects on the Lungs:

Anatomy: Humans Herbal antivirals a pair of lungs in their chests that regulate the average oxygen/carbon dioxide balance throughout over body, a process called respiration. Small hairs-like structures of lungs, which are called the cilia and the basic unit of our lungs, is called the alveoli.

Physiology: Lungs regulate the average oxygen/carbon dioxide balance throughout over body, a process called respiration. Lungs convert the deoxygenated blood coming from the heart into oxygenated blood, which is pumped back into the heart by lungs.

Benefits of HERBAL ANTIVIRALS: Herbal antivirals help to clear the lungs from harmful gasses and toxic material due to its antioxidant capacities. It helps to normalize the healthy pH balance in the lungs and clears the windpipe so that minimal bacteria can enter the respiratory tract. That also helps in clearing our blood directly.

Effects on the heart:

Anatomy: Heart is just as more significant as a fist is. It is a vital organ that helps to regulate the hemodynamics (motion of blood) throughout our body. It has two atria and two ventricles. The heart is supplied by coronary arteries. Pulmonary vessels and vena cava regulate blood to and from the lungs and overall body.

Benefits of HERBAL ANTIVIRALS: Herbal antivirals help to clear the blood, maintains its healthy pH balance, and improves the functional lung capacity. These all help increase the functional capacities of the heart, and thus, proper oxygen balance is maintained throughout the body. Another critical function of herbal antivirals is its lipolytic function. Herbal antivirals are very important in lowering the cholesterol levels of our bodies. That helps in reducing the chances of atherosclerosis and valvular heart diseases. Herbal antivirals help in clearing the coronary arteries, and thus it increases the oxygen supply to the heart is the result of what, the heart works in its maximum capacity. Herbal antivirals are rich in potassium, which is very important in regulating the movement of heart musculature. Heartbeat is regulated by a pacemaker, a bunch of fibers present in our hearts. Potassium is directly linked with the heart rate. If the overall concentration of potassium declines in our body, it causes cardiac arrhythmias, a condition in which heartbeats at a very abnormal pace, and it can be very dangerous. Low potassium levels also indirectly related to fluid accumulation in our bodies called edema. By regulating the potassium levels in our bodies, herbal antivirals can help improve our cardiac and, thus, the general health.

Effects on the liver:

Anatomy: The liver is a capsular structure that is one of the largest organs of the body. Two lobes are present in the liver, and it contains many ligaments. It runs right below the stomach.

Physiology: The liver is called the chemist of the body because the whole chemical taking place in our body is regulated by the liver.

Benefits of HERBAL ANTIVIRALS: Herbal antivirals have some most effective benefits on the liver. Thanks to its buffering and anti-oxidative capacities. Herbal antivirals help to maintain the pH balance of the liver, which is very helpful in the proper functioning of the liver. Herbal antivirals help in the proper production of bile, which is secreted in the liver by the gall bladder and helps in the metabolism of fats. The most crucial benefit of herbal antivirals on liver health is the reduction and prevention of fatty liver. A common illness is known as fatty liver which, accumulates over liver tissue because the liver is unable to metabolize it. The main reason behind this is the overconsumption of fatty food and the inability of the liver and bile to breakdown the fats. Herbal antivirals help in both ways. By regular use of herbal antivirals, dietary habits can be changed as well as less fat gets absorbed from the blood. It reduces the oxidative stress from the liver. Moreover, by its lipolytic pathways, herbal antivirals help the liver to burn more fat and thus reduces the fatty liver. It is essential to know that three grades of fatty liver. First-grade fatty liver can easily be reversed by a low-fat diet, exercise, and using herbal antivirals on a regular basis—Researches Herbal antivirals shown that any abnormality in the liver is directly related to our skin health. By improving the liver capacity, herbal antivirals help to nourish our skin and reduce the risks of acne.

Effects on the Kidney:

Anatomy: kidneys are present in our flank region and posterior to the intestine. They are bean-shaped, and a pair of the kidney is present in humans. The right kidney is lower than the left one because of the presence of the liver.

Physiology: The kidney is the vital organ of our body, and the primary function of the kidney is the formation of urine. Moreover, kidneys indirectly control blood pressure by increasing and decreasing the body's osmotic pressure. This term is associated with the overall water content inside the body. The hormone, which controls the osmotic pressure, is called the Anti-diuretic hormone (ADH).

Benefits of HERBAL ANTIVIRALS: HERBAL ANTIVIRALS has very crucial roles on the health status of our kidneys. First of all, HERBAL ANTIVIRALS is very important in improving the pH of our kidneys, which directly helps in balancing the pH of urine. HERBAL ANTIVIRALS helps in controlling the pH of glomerular filtrate, which is termed as urine by its buffering nature. HERBAL ANTIVIRALS is rich in potassium. This potassium is used by kidneys to be exchanged with sodium through sodium-potassium pumps of kidneys. This helps the dilution of urine by adding more water to it and thus decreases the normal acidic pH of urine. The second most important benefit of HERBAL ANTIVIRALS on kidneys is the detoxification of kidneys. Due to its antioxidant nature, HERBAL ANTIVIRALS helps to clear the kidneys from harmful and damaging free oxygen radicles which are present in abundance in kidneys due to the presence of urea. It helps to relieve the burning sensation of urine as well as helps in the reduction of chances of getting kidney stones. A third most crucial function of HERBAL ANTIVIRALS on kidneys is the prevention of kidney stone formation. Kidney stones are the calcium oxalate crystals which can block the normal glomerular filtrate and thus blockage of urine production to its transportation in ureters and urethra occurs. HERBAL ANTIVIRALS helps to clear the inflammatory mediators, which play a vital role in the formation of calcium oxalate crystals, and it also helps in excretion of these crystals by increasing the water content in urine. Another essential function of HERBAL ANTIVIRALS is the reduction of urea and other nitrogen species such as uric acid crystals from our body by acting on the kidney's filtration capacity. Antioxidant nature of HERBAL ANTIVIRALS helps in reducing the harmful precursors of blood nitrogen from getting stored into the body, and this prevents the chances of gout, which is the acute rise in blood uric acid levels.

CHAPTER7: HERBAL ANTIVIRALS IN PREGNANCY

pregnancy is one of the most amazing miracles of nature, and it comes at the cost of deteriorated health. Fat percentage is increased in pregnancy, which is uncontrollable, but the Herbal antivirals help our stomach and liver to digest or food properly. It reduces the bloating and nausea related to pregnancies.

Cellulitis occurs. Blood pressure and blood glucose levels become uncontrolled. The body becomes more fatty and obese. Nerves get compressed, and edema develops. Skin becomes porous, oily, and becomes prone to acne. Headaches, nausea, morning sickness, and bloating occur. Arthralgia and myalgia happen. Shortness of breath and early fatigue becomes part of pregnancy. Blood becomes depleted, and hemoglobin begins to fall. All these factors require a separate debate because Herbal antivirals are beneficial in all these issues. We will discuss every topic in detail.

Cellulitis:

Cellulitis is the condition in which skin cells become swollen and inflamed. It affects mostly the skin of buttocks, thighs, abdomen, and arm. The cellulitis has a genetic correlation, and it can run in families. Weight reduction after very obese status also leads to unresolved cellulitis. It is also caused by specific skin types. Another critical reason for cellulitis is pregnancy. Herbal antivirals help in the reduction of cellulitis because of its anti-inflammatory results; however, the effects of Herbal antivirals on cellulitis are not validated. Further researches are required, and it is also being noted that only Herbal antivirals are insufficient to overcome the cellulitis issue. A strict low-fat diet, proper high-intensity exercise, and proper hydration are also essential along with regular use of Herbal antivirals.

Acne:

Acne affects almost everyone on earth. It is the accumulation of pus, which is comprised of dead white blood cells and debris of dead bacteria. Low immunity, increase exposure to infections, and diet reduced in essential components can lead to acne issues. The most typical areas of skin that are prone to acne are facial skin. Herbal antivirals very effectively reduce the chances of acne due to its anti-oxidative nature and positive effects on immunity. It also reduces the chances of overproduction of gastric acid, which also causes acne. Moreover, Herbal antivirals help in normalizing the pH of our skin, which leads to fewer acne-related episodes. Another benefit of Herbal antivirals for acne is the reduced production of oil from sebaceous glands of our skin, which is thought to have the most catastrophic effects related to acne issues. This is the reason that oily skin is most prone to acne-related problems. However, regular use of Herbal antivirals and diet rich in protein and antioxidants can help us reduce these episodes.

Dosage: a required dose of Herbal antivirals, 1table spoon of lemon juice, You can use your own face mask by adding Herbal antivirals in the right amount. Add dry ice or pure ice to it. This will make it more stable. Add Aloe Vera gel, two tablespoons of lemon juice, honey two tablespoons, two tablespoons pure glycerin, 10 drops essential oil, and 3-4 tablespoon Herbal organic antivirals. This facial mask will ensure a proper glow and hydration. You can mix four tablespoons of Herbal antivirals in 2 cups of water. Add two tablespoons of lemon juice. Wash your face two times daily, and this will provide a fantastic glow to your skin. This organic face wash is very detoxifying and has the potency to heal skin in no time.

Porous and oily skin:

During pregnancy, sebaceous glands are over-activated, and lipid accumulation in the body causes more production of oil. This leads to acne and porous skin. Herbal antivirals help in reducing the skin oil and making our skin more endure to pregnancy-related issues.

Dosage: you can use a required dose of Herbal antivirals, 1table spoon of lemon juice. You can use your own face mask by adding Herbal antivirals in the right amount. Add dry ice or pure ice to it. This will make it more stable. Add Aloe Vera gel, two tablespoons of lemon juice, honey two tablespoons, two tablespoons pure glycerin, 10 drops essential oil, and 3-4 tablespoon Herbal organic antivirals. This facial mask will ensure a proper glow and hydration. You can mix four tablespoons of Herbal antivirals in 2 cups of water. Add two tablespoons of lemon juice. Wash your face two times daily, and this will provide a fantastic glow to your skin. This organic face wash is very detoxifying and has the potency to heal skin in no time.

Preeclampsia:

It is characterized by an abnormally higher blood pressure range during pregnancy. It can be fatal for both mother and child because if left untreated, it can lead to damage in other vital organs too. It is an emergency during pregnancy and should be addressed as soon as possible. The risk factors of preeclampsia are increased blood cholesterol levels and hormonal disturbances. Herbal antivirals help to reduce blood pressure through its blood regulatory mechanisms, and it also helps in hormonal regulation during pregnancy.

Dosage: a required dose of Herbal antivirals, a 1table spoon of lemon juice, one tablespoon of honey and green tea can also be used. Use it 2/3 times daily.

Pregnancy-related diabetes:

One new type of diabetes is gestational diabetes. This type is prevalent in pregnant women. The most affected period is the second and third trimester. In gestational diabetes, there is an acute rise in blood sugar levels, and it can be dangerous to both mother and child if left untreated. Herbal antivirals are essential to treat gestational diabetes because of the risks of obesity blood glucose levels by increased production of insulin from the pancreas, increase in insulin receptors among liver and other organs, increase in glycolytic pathways increased conversion of glucose into glycogen and increased blood regulation mechanism.

Morning sickness and nausea:

During pregnancy, morning sickness and nausea are two most common feelings for mothers. It is caused by increased overnight production of gastric acid, overproduction of gastric acid and bile, improper digestion of food, and abdominal bloating. Herbal antivirals help in the reduction of morning sickness and nausea to much extent by reducing the overproduction of gastric juice, regulating the basic pH of the body, and suppressing the higher brain center, which senses the nauseated feeling.

Arthralgia and myalgia:

Arthralgia is painful joints, and myalgia is painful muscles. These conditions are prevalent among pregnant females. The most important reason behind these two pathologies is the depletion of essential minerals and vitamins from the body. Pregnancy is a very stressful condition, and additional supplementation of minerals and vitamins should be maintained to prevent any kind of joint or muscle related issue. Herbal antivirals are rich in essential minerals such as calcium, potassium, chromium, zinc, sodium, and magnesium. It is also rich in vitamin A, vitamin B complex, and vitamin C. These ingredients make Herbal antivirals a choice supplement during pregnancy.

Fatigue and shortness of breath:

Early fatigue is the most frequent symptom of pregnancy. Fatigue occurs more frequently as the trimesters' pass. Pregnancy is a very stressful condition, and additional supplementation of minerals and vitamins should be maintained to prevent any kind of joint or muscle related issue. Herbal antivirals are rich in essential minerals such as calcium, potassium, chromium, zinc, sodium, and magnesium. Vitamin A, B complex and vitamin C are frequently present in Herbal antivirals. These ingredients make Herbal antivirals a choice supplement during pregnancy. Shortness of breath is another condition. Increased water content in the lungs and increased weight with reduced hemoglobin stores of blood causes oxidative stress to a pregnant body, which leads to shortness of breath. Herbal antivirals help in thermoregulation, regulation of blood flow and hemoglobin, and this helps in reducing the episodes of shortness of breath.

Headaches and nerve entrapment:

Headache associated with pregnancy is caused by severe oxidative stress and reduced stores of vitamins and minerals. Arthralgia and myalgia, increased blood pressure, poor blood sugar control, fatigue, and shortness of breath lead to headaches and dizziness in pregnancy. Herbal antivirals, with its rich characteristics, help in the reduction of headaches and dizziness.

During pregnancy, the body becomes edematous, and the water content of the body increases to many folds. Herbal antivirals help in the regulation of the water content of the body and reduce edema, which is the main reason behind nerve entrapments during pregnancy.

CHAPTER 8: HERBAL ANTIVIRALS FOR CHILDREN

Children have a very delicate body. Infants can also use herbal medicine, but the route of administration, as well as dosing, can be very troublesome to decide. A full cup of tea and an ice cube of decoction is a terrible idea when used for infants. We Herbal antivirals to decide the safest routes of administration because of the delicate body of infants. Breast milk is a natural source to nourish babies from the nutrients in the mother's blood. Breast milk is the safest from all the routes of nourishment because many complex nutrients that cannot be introduced in an infant's body otherwise can easily be inserted through breast milk. A mother and her child, both can be benefited in that way. Some herbal medicines are really infant friendly while others can be harsher on the delicate infant body, so a careful consideration before administration is essential to avoid any kind of side effects. Another significant benefit is to insert potent herbal antibacterial medicine inside an infant to make more him/her more immune with side effects of getting sick from antibacterials is to introduce them from the mother's breast milk. It will boost the natural immunization responses in both mother and her infant.

Precautions for children:

1. Don't use concentrated medicine on children.
2. Never use bitter tasted medicine for infants
3. Herbal medicine can cause gut issues in children, so the dose must be well calculated.

4. Keep all types of herbal medicine away from the reach of children

5. If any sign of toxicity occurs, seek expert medical advice immediately.

6. Mothers should have the necessary training to use herbal medicine for their newborns and children.

CHAPTER: HERBAL ANTIVIRALS FOR OLD AGE:

Herbal medicine is highly essential for the old age population because it can fight many infections as well as can boost the immunity of the body. It can provide many benefits for the fragile skeleton of the old age population. However, some specific precautions are highly necessary to follow when administrating herbal antivirals in the old age population.

1. Don't use concentrated medicine on Old age population.
2. Herbal medicine can cause gut issues in the old age population, so the dose must be well calculated.
3. If any sign of toxicity occurs, seek expert medical advice immediately.
4. Caregivers should have the necessary training in using herbal medicine for the old age population.
5. Old patients may have many illnesses together, so a calculated dose for every illness is highly essential to avoid toxicity.
6. The medicine should be labeled for the convenience of old patients.

SIDE EFFECTS OF HERBAL ANTIVIRALS:

A balanced and well-calculated dose of herbal antivirals cannot hurt, but too much consumption of herbal antivirals can lead to side effects. After all, excess of everything is terrible. Some most typical side effects are discussed below:

Delayed stomach emptying:

People with type 1 diabetes suffer from a condition called gastroparesis. As the name implies, gastro is related to stomach, and paresis is a medical term related to the weakness of nerves. In type 1 diabetes, nerves of the stomach are unable to effectively process the food and cause delayed emptying of the stomach. In this condition, herbal antivirals should not be used because it can further increase the problem because of its satiety effects. Researches showed that adding only two tablespoons of herbal antivirals can cause the delayed emptying of the stomach. The sign and symptoms of gastroparesis are nausea, feeling of fullness, and flatulence.

Digestive issues:

Some people are intolerant to acids, and hence, herbal antivirals contain acetic acid, its use can further increase the problem. Herbal antivirals increase the feeling of fullness, and if a person with early satiety disorder consumes herbal antivirals, it can cause digestive issues.

Low blood potassium levels:

Herbal antivirals contain a small amount of potassium, but the higher doses of herbal antivirals can lead to the reverse mechanism of the body in which excess potassium is being excreted, and it can lead to low blood potassium levels. It can prove fatal because potassium is the main mineral in the regulation of heart rate.

Low calcium levels:

Increased potassium levels come in the cost of decreased calcium levels. So, the overuse of herbal antivirals can lead to low calcium levels in our bodies.

Osteoporosis and osteopenia:

Osteopenia is decreased bone mineral density, and if it is present with one or more fractures, it is termed as osteoporosis. Osteoporosis means porous bones, i.e., calcium levels, are drastically decreased. A case study showed that too much consumption of herbal antivirals for an extended period of time leads to osteoporosis inpatient because the buffer systems had to act against the high acidic medium of blood, which came in the cost of calcium and potassium exchange from the body.

Erosion of tooth enamel:

Enamel is a protective layer on our teeth, which prevents discoloration. Enamel is intolerant to acidic nature, and thus too much herbal antivirals can cause erosion of tooth enamel. This leads to discoloration of teeth.

Sore throat:

Sore throat is a condition that is caused by a variety of factors, and acidic exposure is one of them. If the esophagus is too sensitive or too much herbal antivirals are used, it can lead to a sore throat. However, a balanced amount of herbal antivirals can prevent sore throat by decreasing peptic acid production.

Skin burns:

Herbal antivirals can cause erosion of skin surface in sensitive skin. However, this effect is not clearly understood. It is believed that too much acidic exposure can lead to decreased pH of the skin, which leads to its erosion.

Adverse interaction with drugs:

Herbal antivirals have the potency to interact with various drugs

In diabetic patients, it can interact with insulin or glucose-lowering drugs and thus leads to drastically low blood sugar levels in patients with high blood pressure, herbal antivirals can interact with diuretics and can cause increased excretion of potassium, and hence hypokalemia can occur.

In patients on potassium lowering drugs, excessive use of herbal antivirals can lead to a drastic lowering of blood potassium levels.

Summary:

This is the end of our book on herbal antivirals. All the essential details about the basics, formation, use, and benefits of herbal antivirals have been covered in detail. This book will provide in-depth insight into herbal medicine for beginners and advanced herbalists to know the core of herbalism art of practice.